NCA
Review for
the Clinical
Laboratory
Sciences

NCA REVIEW FOR THE CLINICAL LABORATORY SCIENCES

Second Edition

Edited by
Sharon L. Zablotney, Ph.D., CLS
Associate Dean, College of Natural Science, and Professor of Medical Technology and Microbiology, Michigan State University, East Lansing

Associate Editors
Joan E. Aldrich, M.S., CLS/C
Assistant Professor, Department of Medical Laboratory Sciences, University of Texas Southwestern Medical Center, Dallas; Chairman, Chemistry Committee of NCA, Washington, D.C.

Susan J. Beck, M.S., CLS
Assistant Professor, Division of Medical Technology, University of North Carolina, Chapel Hill; Chairman, Immunohematology and Immunology Committee of NCA, Washington, D.C.

Susanne W. Conner, M.A., CLS, CLDir
Education Coordinator, Cooperative Medical Technology Program, and Laboratory Safety Officer, The Children's Hospital Medical Center of Akron, Ohio; Chairman, Laboratory Practice Committee of NCA, Washington, D.C.

Holly K. Hall, M.A., CLS
Assistant Professor and Clinical Director, Department of Medical Technology, College and Allied Health Professions, University of South Alabama, Mobile; Chairman, Microbiology Committee of NCA, Washington, D.C.

Elizabeth B. Sawyer, B.S., CLS
Medical Teaching Technologist, Microbiology, University of South Alabama Medical Center, Mobile

Marian Schwabbauer, M.A., CLS, CLSp (H)
Program Director, Clinical Laboratory Sciences, University of Iowa, Iowa City; Chairman, Hematology Committee of NCA, Washington, D.C.

Little, Brown and Company
Boston/Toronto/London

This is a second edition of *The NCA Review for the Clinical Laboratory Sciences*, edited by **James L. Bender.**

Second Printing

Copyright © 1989 by National Certification Agency for Medical Laboratory Personnel

Second Edition

Previous edition copyright © 1985 by National Certification Agency for Medical Laboratory Personnel

Library of Congress Catalog Card No. 89-80154

ISBN 0-316-59925-5

Printed in the United States of America

EB

Contents

Preface to the Second Edition

The NCA Review for the Clinical Laboratory Sciences was developed to assist candidates preparing for certification and recertification examinations. This second edition of the study guide is a restructuring of the previous edition in that it divides the six chapters of the book, including the study test, into sections specific to the knowledge requirements for CLT and CLS certification. Candidates at both these career entry levels will find this new format time-saving and efficient.

As in the first edition, the study questions of the first five sections are accompanied by a list of possible answers, followed by the correct choice and an explanation for the selection. A compilation of pertinent reference materials is found at the end of each section. Lastly, the Review Tests section offers a sampling of items representative of the actual CLS and CLT certification exams; an answer key follows each test, kept separate for a more reliable personal assessment of knowledge.

I would like to thank the thousands of laboratory professionals who have supported NCA and the peer-review certification process.

S. L. Z.

Preface to the First Edition

NCA Review for the Clinical Laboratory Sciences was developed to assist candidates preparing for the CLS certification and recertification examinations. The test items included in the review areas and sample test are comparable to, and representative of, the items used in the certifying examinations. Although mastering the questions in this review book does not ensure that a candidate will pass the certification or recertification examination, it should help the candidate to identify areas of weakness that may be strengthened by additional study and review. By using the methods suggested in the introduction, candidates can become more familiar with the competency-based philosophy of certification, the basis for establishing the pass score, the type and content of characteristic test items, and test-taking strategies.

An important feature of this review book is the explanation accompanying each item, which discusses the rationale for the correct response. This enhances the effectiveness of the book as a study tool. We recommend that candidates review each item section in depth before taking the sample test in the last section of this book. The items in the sample test represent both the type and mix of items used in the actual certification examination. The answer key is provided separately so that the experience with the sample test can truly be one of self-assessment.

Many people have contributed their time to make this review possible. I am especially indebted to the following: Patricia Amos, M.S., for the introduction; the associate editors; the people who submitted the items and explanations in each discipline, listed at the opening of each chapter; and the NCA staff in Washington, D.C.

The NCA has made significant strides since its inception. Use of a competency-based, criterion-referenced instrument to establish a basis for certification has attained increasing acceptance in the laboratory-science community. This review represents the efforts of a large volunteer segment of the clinical laboratory science profession, which has shown it is prepared to define its scope of practice and to determine the standards that must be met to enter that practice. We commend those who are concerned enough about such standards to use this book.

J. L. B.

Introduction

Patricia A. Amos

The NCA certification examinations for clinical laboratory technicians (CLT) and clinical laboratory scientists (CLS) are designed to assess the examinee's ability to function with competence in a clinical laboratory as an entry-level practitioner. A generalist examination and categorical examinations in the disciplines of chemistry, hematology, immunohematology, and microbiology are offered twice each year throughout the United States. This review book is designed to prepare a candidate to pass CLT- and CLS-level examinations by explaining (1) the examination content and format, and method for establishing the pass score, (2) the types and content of test items found on the exams, and (3) test-taking strategies. Careful review of this material should assist the candidate in pinpointing areas of weakness that can be strengthened through additional study and in increasing his or her ability to do well on the examination.

CONTENT, FORMAT, SCORING

Examination Content

The NCA examinations are designed to be job-related. The test items have been derived from career-entry statements of competence developed by the American Society for Medical Technology. These statements identify what a laboratory scientist should know and be able to do on entering the field. The test items measure performance in the following categories:

Request for test performance
Specimen collection
Specimen preparation
Reagent preparation/contents
Instrumentation and equipment
Maintenance and safety
Quality assurance
Theory/principles
Tests/procedures
Clinical correlations
Significant parameters

The subject classifications within each of the five major areas represented on the generalist examination are:

Chemistry
Carbohydrates
Lipids
Proteins/enzymes
Nonprotein nitrogen
Electrolytes/acids and bases/gases
Toxicology
Endocrinology/vitamins
Heme synthesis and degradation
Body fluids other than blood, serum, and urine

Techniques
Renal anatomy/physiology/tests
Urinalysis

Hematology/Hemostasis
Blood origin/development/function
Morphology of blood cells
Laboratory methods
Cytochemistry
RBC disorders
WBC disorders
Theory/methods
Disease states/correlations

Immunohematology/Immunology
Cellular and humoral immunity
Immunoglobulins Complement
Laboratory methods
Serology/pregnancy testing
Donor selection/collection
Blood systems
Antibody testing
Transfusion therapy/reaction
Hemolytic anemia
Blood storage and handling

Microbiology
Cocci and other positive rods
Enterics and other negative rods
Bacteriology—miscellaneous
Anaerobes
Procedures
Mycology
Parasitology
Virology/rickettsiae/chlamydiae
Antimicrobial agents/studies
Infection control/environmental studies*

Laboratory Practice
Safety
Mathematics and statistics
Instrumentation
Quality control
Specimen handling
Education*
Management*

*CLS examination only

Laws/regulations
Records and reporting systems

The test items on an NCA examination are selected to cover the range of cognitive abilities from "recall" to "evaluation." Using the classification defined by Bloom, these abilities include:

Knowledge: the ability to remember (recall) ideas, facts, or phenomena
Comprehension: the ability to make use of an idea being communicated, without necessarily relating it to other material or seeing its fullest implications
Application: the ability to use abstractions in the form of general ideas, rules of procedures, or generalized methods
Analysis: the ability to break down ideas into their constituent elements, such that the relative hierarchy of ideas is made clear
Evaluation: the ability to make judgments about the value of materials and methods for given purposes.

Examination Formats

The major difference between the generalist examination for CLT and CLS is in the content and level of practice tested. The CLS certification test recognizes persons capable of developing and evaluating laboratory procedures using a high degree of independent judgment. Persons who have completed a baccalaureate program in the clinical laboratory sciences or who have the requisite combination of education and experience (as defined in eligibility requirements) should take the CLS examination.

The CLT certification recognizes the person whose primary responsibilities relate to the performance of specific laboratory procedures under supervision. People who have graduated from an accredited laboratory education program, possess a certificate of military laboratory specialist, or have the requisite work experience (as defined in eligibility requirements) should take the CLT examination.

The generalist CLS examination and the categorical CLS examinations differ in the number of items and the content:

	Type of test		
	Generalist (CLS)	Generalist (CLT)	Categorical
Distribution (no.)			
Hematology	40	40	40 in one of the
Chemistry	40	40	subject specialties
Immunohematology	40	40	
Microbiology	40	40	
Lab practice	40	40	40
Total	200	200	80 (plus 40 for each additional subject attempted)

	Type of test		
	Generalist (CLS)	Generalist (CLT)	Categorical
Level of question (%)			
Knowledge/ comprehension	25	85	25
Application	50	15	50
Analysis/evaluation	25	0	25

Scoring the Examination

Performance Standards

The NCA examinations identify persons who demonstrate the ability to perform at the minimal level of competence as defined by the professional organization. This "minimum competency" approach does not rank examinees; rather, it serves to ensure that persons granted certificates are capable of performing the tasks necessary for satisfactory job performance. The examinations are, therefore, criterion-referenced.

The passing score for these examinations is defined as the level at which a minimally competent person performs. In establishing a passing score for the examinations, NCA considers the following two factors:

The passing score must reflect the minimum skill level actually required for successful job performance.
The passing score must not adversely affect groups of people defined by specific cultural characteristics.

The consequences of classification errors are clearly serious. If a candidate possesses the skills necessary for successful job performance, but, by error, receives a failing grade, his or her career might suffer. On the other hand, if a candidate does not possess the required skills but receives a passing grade, his or her job performance might adversely affect others. Every effort is made, therefore, to classify examinees correctly as competent or not competent to perform as a clinical laboratory scientist or clinical laboratory technician.

Procedure for Establishing a Pass Score

Expert practitioners, who are chosen for their knowledge of an area within the clinical laboratory science field (e.g., clinical microbiology) and for their experience with practitioners at career-entry, review examination items. Independent of one another, they determine the percentage of minimally competent persons who would be able to answer each question correctly. The "expected" percentages for each item are averaged to give a criterion score for the item. The criterion scores for all test items included are used to determine the pass score for an examination.

Each item contributes one point to the final test score in an "anonymous" manner. This means that an examinee does not need to answer a specific set of items correctly but must answer correctly at least as many items as the pass score. For example, in order to pass a 200-item test with a pass score of 120, an examinee may correctly answer any combination of items as long as at least 120 of them are answered correctly.

To further calibrate the variation between test administrations, the raw scores are equated to a fixed-scale score. This passing scaled score is held constant across all test administrations.

TYPES AND CONTENT OF TEST ITEMS

Types of Test Items

Most test items are of the multiple-choice type, consisting of a statement or question and four alternative answers, only one of which is correct. Some items require the "best" answer; that is, although an incorrect response may be partially true, the correct response is clearly better. Only correct answers contribute to the total score; no points are subtracted for incorrect answers or items not answered. Standardized current nomenclature is used:

Microbiology: Microorganisms are named according to the taxonomy of the Centers for Disease Control, HEW Publication CDC 83-56, 1977 Taxonomic Nomenclature Changes in Enterobacteriaceae.
Hematology: Système Internationale Units are used for hematologic data.

Examples of Test Items

Multiple Choice—One "Best" Answer

EXAMPLE:

The quality control data for normal and abnormal ranges for hemoglobin determinations, erythrocyte counts, and hematocrit values have been acceptable for the last 4 days. A patient sample on day 5 gives the following results:

WBC: 17.5×10^9/L   Hct: 0.381 L/L   MCHC: 43.3 g/dl
RBC: 4.12×10^{12}/L   MCV: 90 fl
HGB: 16.5 g/dl   MCH: 39.0 pg

The protocol to follow to obtain precise and accurate results as economically as possible is to

    A. Check the peripheral blood smear; if the results correlate, report patient data to the physician.
    B. Repeat normal and abnormal hematocrit controls; if the results are acceptable report patient data.
  *C. Observe the plasma; if it appears to be lipemic or icteric, prepare a plasma bank to correct the whole-blood hemoglobin.
    D. Recalculate the indices since they are in error.

TEST-TAKING STRATEGIES

Most people feel an increasing amount of apprehension as the date for a certification examination approaches. Such anxiety is natural and desirable, since feeling overly confident can dull the initiative to prepare adequately for the exam. On the other hand, undue anxiety can result in a score that does not reflect true ability. The following suggestions, none of them novel, might be used as a guide to stimulate the optimal degree of confidence to perform well.

Before the Examination
Study
There can be no substitute for knowing the subject matter. This book illustrates both the scope and the depth of the questions and should be thoroughly reviewed.

Practice Answering Techniques
The strategy for typical multiple-choice items is rather straightforward. After carefully reading the *complete* question and *all* alternative responses, select the most nearly correct response. If the correct response is not obvious, eliminate (by marking the examination booklet), the wrong responses one by one and then guess from the remaining responses.

The strategy for matching-multiple choice items is similar. Mark the "matches" that are obvious and guess the remainder.

Organize
Be sure to have the full address of the test site. Allow plenty of time for arrival (and parking the car, if necessary). Take the test administration card, two #2 pencils, and a watch (other materials are not necessary).

Calculators
The use of calculators on NCA examinations is neither needed nor allowed. The development of small programmable calculators has created difficulty in ensuring test security as well as controlling cheating. Therefore, items featured on an examination involve only the identification of the formula to be used for analyzing the data presented or simple mathematical calculations that do not require use of a calculator.

Get a Good Night's Sleep
Try to approach the examination well rested. People perform better when they are refreshed than when they are fatigued.

During the Examination
Read the Directions and Questions
Before the examination begins, you will have time to check that you have the correct booklet and test form. Read the directions on the booklet cover. After the test begins, be sure you read the questions carefully. An important element in careful question reading is not to read more into the question than is actually there. NCA questions have been written and reviewed to state precisely what is meant. *Reading directions and questions carefully is the most important factor identified by students achieving high scores on tests.*

Scan the Examination First
Take a few minutes to quickly look over the entire examination. This will give you an overall view of what to expect as well as a check that no pages of the

booklet are missing. The overall view will allow you to take the next step—developing a timetable.

Develop a Timetable

You will have 4 hours to complete the CLS examination, which consists of 200 questions. This allows you 1 minute, 20 seconds per answer. Answer the easier questions first. Never spend too much time on any one item. After you have finished the less difficult questions, go back to the more difficult ones. This process will allow you extra time to spend on the harder questions. *Keep your cool;* don't fight the examination. There is nothing you can do to change the test once you receive it. If there are questions you feel are unfair, don't waste time getting angry. All examinees must deal with the same "unreasonable" questions. If you feel a question is especially unfair, report your feelings to NCA after the exam.

Watch out for Skipping on the Answer Sheet

Be sure you are marking on the answer sheet the same number you are reading in the test booklet. Nothing is so annoying as to realize you are reading question 90 and marking answer 89, and you don't know which answer you skipped. You might have to go back to the beginning, and the loss of time could be disastrous.

Draw a Blank? Don't Panic!

If you "freeze" or "block" on any item or group of items, don't panic. A temporary lapse of memory is a normal phenomenon. Simply move on and come back to the question later. The more anxious you become, the more you will inhibit your performance. In examination situations, calmness and alertness are your assets.

Guess When Necessary

Since there is no penalty for marking a wrong answer, you should answer every question. Even if you know nothing about a subject, you have a 25% chance of guessing the answer. However, if you have partial knowledge about the subject, which is likely since you had to meet the NCA eligibility requirements to take the examination, you can improve your chance of guessing the right answer by eliminating those distractors you know to be wrong.

Changing Your Answers

Generally it is better not to change an answer because first impressions are usually correct. However, if you misread a question originally or recall some information not previously remembered, or another question on the test jogs your memory about some relevant fact, you may improve your score by changing your answer.

Realistic Expectations

No one ever made a perfect score on a major standardized examination. In clinical laboratory science, as in other fields, the certifying examination can only sample the subjects addressed in the educational program or used on the job. Therefore, when you are faced with questions for which you don't know or are not sure about the answers, mark down an answer or leave a blank and come back later, but don't get upset. Everyone will miss some questions. However, a calm and positive attitude will permit you to continue without anxiety or interference with the questions that follow.

In summary, there is no substitute for knowing the content on an examination. Nor is there a substitute for a good understanding of the process involved in taking an examination. Both content knowledge and the ability to take examinations successfully can be improved by study and practice.

NCA
Review for
the Clinical
Laboratory
Sciences

Section Editor
Joan E. Aldrich, M.S.

Contributors
Kathleen J. Clayson, M.S.
Diane Coiner, M.S.
Janet Noecker
Robert S. Putnam, M.D.

Qutub T. Ali, M.S.
Sue G. Barr, M.S.
Kathleen Becan-McBride, Ed.D.
Eileen Carreiro-Lewandowski, M.S.
V. Michele Chenault, M.A.
Christine Carter, M.S.
Susan Cockayne, M.S.
Janet Duben-Von Laufen, M.S.
Gary Gill
Patricia A. Hemmerle, M.S.
Jessie Hansen, M.S.
Jean Holter, Ed.D.
Ruthann Hyduke
Sharon A. Jackson, M.Ed.
Christine King, M.S.
Robert L. Klick, M.S.
William J. Korzun, M.S.
Deborah Kullerd-Smith, M.P.H.
Sharon M. Miller, Ph.C.
Barbara Minderman
Fulvantiben D. Mistry, Ph.D.
Ruth E. Morris, M.Ed.
Robert E. Moore, Ph.D.
Karen E. Myers, M.A.
Margaret L. Nance, M.Ed.
Sharon Parker, Ph.D.
Glenda D. Price, Ph.D.
Virginia Randolph, M.A.
Carla E. Salmon
Larry Schoeff, M.S.
Anne M. Sullivan, M.S.
M. Gaye Tison
Janet L. Zins, Ph.D.

CLT Review Questions

1. In an adult, a blood glucose level of 35 mg/dl is

    A. Dangerously high
    B. Dangerously low
    C. Normal
    D. Physiologically impossible

The answer is B. True hypoglycemia of this magnitude can cause neurologic symptoms and may result in irreversible damage. A very low serum glucose value also may be an artifact caused by cellular metabolism or bacterial contamination if serum is not separated from cells promptly. (Tietz, p. 440; Kaplan and Pesce, p. 727)

2. The hexokinase reaction for serum glucose

    A. Reduces cupric ions to cuprous ions
    B. Measures the amount of hydrogen peroxide produced
    C. Uses a glucose-6-phosphate dehydrogenase (G-6-PD)–catalyzed indicator reaction
    D. Produces a green condensation product with o-toluidine

The answer is C. Hexokinase catalyzes the phosphorylation of several monosaccharides using ATP as the phosphate donor and producing the corresponding sugar-6-phosphate. The G-6-PD–catalyzed indicator reaction uses only glucose-6-phosphate as substrate. The high specificity of this latter reaction prevents interference from other monosaccharides. (Tietz, p. 427; Kaplan and Pesce, p. 1033; Bishop et al., p. 301)

3. Which of the glucose tolerances shown in the figure on p. 3 meet NDDG (National Diabetes Data Group) criteria for the diagnosis of diabetes mellitus?

    A. Curves 1 and 2
    B. Curves 1 and 4
    C. Curves 3 and 4
    D. Only curve 4

The answer is C. NDDG criteria for the diagnosis of diabetes mellitus include either (1) fasting serum glucose level greater than 140 mg/dl on more than one occasion, or (2) two or more serum samples with glucose levels greater than 200 mg/dl following a meal. Curve 3 meets the latter criterion and curve 4 meets both criteria. (Tietz, p. 433; Kaplan and Pesce, p. 544; Bishop et al., p. 304)

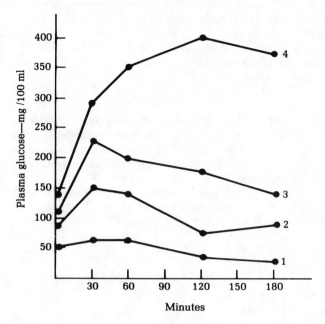

(Tietz, 1976, p. 252)

4. A lipemic serum has an elevated level of

   A. Cholesterol
   B. HDL
   C. Phospholipid
   D. Triglycerides

The answer is D. Lipemia is the result of light scattering by large fat-containing micelles. Both chylomicrons and VLDL particles have large enough diameters to cause this effect and both of them contain a high proportion of triglycerides. (Tietz, p. 457; Kaplan and Pesce, p. 576; Bishop et al., pp. 348, 353)

5. An enzymatic method for measuring cholesterol in serum uses the reduced form of a dye and all of these reagents *except*

   A. Cholesterol esterase
   B. Cholesterol oxidase
   C. NADH
   D. Peroxidase

The answer is C. The enzymatic method for measuring total cholesterol incubates serum with cholesterol esterase (to release free cholesterol), cholesterol oxidase (to oxidize cholesterol and produce hydrogen peroxide), and a reduced dye which is oxidized to a chromogen by hydrogen peroxide and peroxidase. (Tietz, p. 474; Kaplan and Pesce, p. 1195; Bishop et al., p. 355)

6. pH 8.6 is used for serum protein electrophoresis so that

   A. All serum proteins will have a net negative charge
   B. All serum proteins will have a net positive charge
   C. Electroendosmosis is avoided
   D. Heat production is minimized

The answer is A. Proteins are ampholytes whose terminal amino and carboxyl groups, as well as ionizable side groups on component amino acids, change their charges with change in pH. At a pH higher than the pK of these ionizable groups, dissociable hydrogen ions are lost to the medium resulting in no charge on each amino group and a negative charge on each carboxyl group. The net charge on the protein therefore becomes negative. The amount of heat produced and the buffer migration (electroendosmosis) which occur are determined in large part by the concentration of the buffer. (Tietz, pp. 77–78; Kaplan and Pesce, p. 1309; Bishop et al., p. 185)

7. Biuret reagent reacts with

   A. Ammonia released from proteins
   B. Free amino groups in proteins
   C. Peptide bonds in proteins
   D. Tyrosine residues in proteins

The answer is C. In alkaline solution, cuprous ions in biuret reagent form coordinate bonds with the carbonyl groups of peptide bonds resulting in a colored complex. (Tietz, p. 315; Kaplan and Pesce, p. 1316; Bishop et al., p. 181)

8. Which one of these protein bands, when separated from serum by electrophoresis on cellulose acetate, contains only one protein?

   A. Albumin
   B. Alpha$_1$-globulin
   C. Alpha$_2$-globulin
   D. Beta-globulin

The answer is A. The large peak of albumin seen on a serum electropherogram is virtually pure albumin. Since electrophoresis on cellulose acetate separates proteins according to their net charges, the other peaks seen are mixtures of the proteins which share approximately the same net charge. (Tietz, p. 313; Kaplan and Pesce, pp. 1312–1313)

9. Which serum isoenzyme result may be falsely increased if a hemolyzed sample is analyzed?

   A. CK-MB (CK-2)
   B. CK-MM (CK-3)
   C. LD isoenzyme 1 (HHHH)
   D. LD isoenzyme 2 (MMMM)

The answer is C. Erythrocytes are rich in LD isoenzyme 1. Hemolysis, whether artifactual or in vivo, can cause LD isoenzyme 1 to be increased and the LD-isoenzyme-1–to–LD-isoenzyme-2 ratio to exceed 1.0. The data then may be indistinguishable from those obtained following myocardial infarction. Erythrocytes do not contain a discernible amount of LD isoenzyme 5 nor any isoenzyme of creatine kinase. (Tietz, p. 384; Kaplan and Pesce, pp. 1119, 1129; Bishop et al., pp. 217–218)

10. Which enzyme catalyzes this reaction?

   L-alanine + 2-oxoglutarate→L-glutamate + pyruvate

   A. Alkaline phosphatase
   B. Alanine aminotransferase (ALT)
   C. Aspartate aminotransferase (AST)
   D. Gamma-glutamyl transpeptidase (GGT)

The answer is B. The rules for trivial enzyme names state that the first name of an enzyme indicates its substrate and the second name indicates the type of reaction catalyzed. Thus, in this case, alanine is the principal substrate and transamination between alanine and the general substrate oxoglutarate is the reaction catalyzed by ALT. (Tietz, p. 370; Kaplan and Pesce, p. 1088; Bishop et al., p. 220)

11. Which of these serum samples is satisfactory for acid phosphatase measurement?

   A. Acidified to pH 5
   B. Heated to 56° C for 30 min
   C. Hemolyzed
   D. Refrigerated for 18 hr

The answer is A. Acid phosphatase in serum is very unstable. At a pH below 5.4 or when frozen, the enzyme activity is stabilized. Erythrocytes contain large amounts of acid phosphatase and make a hemolyzed sample unsatisfactory for the analysis. (Tietz, p. 409; Kaplan and Pesce, p. 1082; Bishop et al., p. 224)

12. Turbidimetric assays for serum lipase measure the

   A. Amount of bile acid produced
   B. Amount of titratable acid produced
   C. Rate of degradation of triglycerides
   D. Rate of production of NADH

The answer is C. Lipase acts at the surface of nonwater-soluble triglyceride micelles, hydrolyzing terminal fatty acids from glycerol. As the micelles become smaller they scatter less light and the substrate suspension becomes less turbid. The rate of clearing of turbidity reflects the amount of lipase activity. (Tietz, pp. 400–401; Kaplan and Pesce, p. 1131; Bishop et al., p. 228)

13. Urease hydrolyzes urea to form

    A. Ammonia
    B. An amino acid
    C. Creatinine
    D. NADH

The answer is A. Urease is a plant enzyme that breaks down urea into ammonia and CO_2. These products then form an equilibrium in aqueous solution with ammonium and carbonate ions. (Tietz, p. 677; Kaplan and Pesce, p. 1258; Bishop et al., p. 413)

14. Increased serum uric acid is found in all *except*

    A. Gout
    B. Hypothyroidism
    C. Lesch-Nyhan syndrome
    D. Renal failure

The answer is B. Thyroid hormones have no specific effect on formation of uric acid. Gout is the disease caused by deposition of excessive uric acid in body spaces, e.g., joints. Lesch-Nyhan syndrome is a rare inborn error of metabolism in which the salvage enzyme of purine catabolism is deficient. This results in excessive production of the purine catabolite uric acid. Renal failure results in inability to clear the blood of waste products including uric acid. (Tietz, pp. 685, 696; Kaplan and Pesce, pp. 418, 717, 856; Bishop et al., p. 417)

15. Ionized calcium should be measured using a sample which is

    A. Anticoagulated with EDTA
    B. Deproteinized
    C. Protected from oxidation
    D. The same pH as the patient's blood

The answer is D. Calcium is present in blood in three forms: free ionized calcium, protein-bound calcium, and nonionized calcium salts. Only the ionized form is physiologically active. The dissociation of calcium from its complexed forms depends on pH. This is particularly true of protein-bound calcium since hydrogen ions and calcium ions, both being cations, compete for binding sites on protein. A change in the pH of the blood sample would alter the amount of calcium bound to protein and therefore alter the amount of free ionized calcium measured. (Tietz, pp. 705, 717; Kaplan and Pesce, p. 1052; Bishop et al., p. 275)

16. Identify the results that *are not* in electrolyte balance. (Results are in mmol/L.)

	Na^+	K^+	Cl^-	CO_2 content
A.	125	4.5	100	10
B.	135	3.5	95	28
✓ C.	145	4.0	90	15
D.	150	5.0	110	30

The answer is C. Electrolyte balance is judged by calculating the anion gap: (Na + K) − (CL + CO_2 content). The difference reflects the net concentration of anions that have not been included in the equation. Anion gap is normally 10 to 20 mmol/L. (Tietz, pp. 665–666; Kaplan and Pesce, p. 1044; Bishop et al., p. 285)

17. Osmolality is proportional to

    A. Activity of ions per kilogram of solvent
    B. Grams of solute per kilogram of solvent
 ✓ C. Moles of dissolved solute per kilogram of solvent
    D. Mass of solute per kilogram of solvent

The answer is C. Osmolality expresses the total effective concentration of all solutes. The osmotic pressure of a solution is determined by the total number of solute particles per volume of solvent irrespective of whether the particles are ions or nonionized solutes. (Tietz, p. 101; Kaplan and Pesce, p. 1070; Bishop et al., p. 265)

18. Flame emission spectrophotometry for analysis of sodium and potassium uses a sample diluted with a lithium solution for all of these reasons *except*

    A. Lithium is required to ionize sodium and potassium salts.
    B. Lithium emission responds to variations in the sample aspiration rate.
    C. Lithium is excited and emits light in the same temperature range as sodium and potassium.
    D. Lithium minimizes error due to mutual excitation.

The answer is A. Virtually all sodium and potassium salts ionize spontaneously in aqueous solution. Lithium is added to samples for flame emission analysis of sodium and potassium so that it can act as an internal standard and a radiation buffer. These functions are defined by answers B, C, and D. (Tietz, p. 63; Kaplan and Pesce, p. 65; Bishop, et al., p. 97)

19. Which formula gives the best estimate of the expected value for serum osmolality? (Electrolyte results are in mmol/L; glucose and BUN results are in mg/dL.)

    A. $2.5 \times Na^+$
    B. $Na^+ + K^+ + Cl^- + CO_2$ content
    C. $(1.86 \times Na^+) + (1/18 \times glucose) + (1/2.8 \times BUN) + 9$
    D. $(Na^+ + K^+) − (Cl^- + CO_2$ content)

The answer is C. Sodium is by far the major cation in serum, and there is an anion for each cation. Thus $2 \times$ Na (in mmol/L) accounts for most ions present, although empirically the factor 1.86 fits observed values better. Dividing glucose (in mg/dl) by 18 and BUN in (mg/dl) by 2.8 converts these values to their millimolar equivalents. The remaining constituents in serum normally amount to 9 mmol/L. (Tietz, pp. 666–667; Kaplan and Pesce, p. 234; Bishop et al., p. 266)

20. The normal ratio of bicarbonate ion to carbonic acid in arterial blood is

    A. 0.03:1
    B. 1:1.8
  ✓ C. 20:1
    D. 6.1:7.4

The answer is C. The Henderson-Hasselbalch equation defines the ratio of base to acid that is required for a given pH. At normal arterial pH the ratio of concentrations of bicarbonate ion to carbonic acid is 20:1. The pKa of this buffer system in whole blood at 37°C is 6.1. (Tietz, p. 649; Kaplan and Pesce, p. 389; Bishop et al., p. 245)

21. Which of these patients has respiratory acidosis?

	Arterial blood pH	Arterial pCO_2
A.	Decreased	Decreased
✓ B.	Decreased	Increased
C.	Increased	Decreased
D.	Increased	Increased

The answer is B. Respiratory acidosis is defined as decreased blood pH caused by an absolute excess of CO_2. The excess CO_2 relative to bicarbonate concentration causes blood pH to decrease. (Tietz, pp. 657–659; Kaplan and Pesce, p. 400; Bishop et al., pp. 245–246)

22. The toxic effects of carbon monoxide are caused by

    A. Displacement of oxygen from heme
    B. Formation of methemoglobin
    C. Oxidation of heme iron
    D. A right-shifted oxyhemoglobin dissociation curve

The answer is A. Carbon monoxide strongly binds to heme at the same site that oxygen does and prevents formation of oxyhemoglobin. The iron in the heme pocket remains in its active ferrous state. When oxygen gradually displaces carbon monoxide from carboxyhemoglobin, the function of the hemoglobin molecule is restored. (Tietz, p. 885; Kaplan and Pesce, p. 621; Bishop et al., p. 550)

23. A blood sample for routine therapeutic drug monitoring is usually obtained

    A. At the calculated peak time after a dose
    B. Just after a dose is administered
    ✓C. Just before the next scheduled dose trough
    D. One half-life after a dose is administered

The answer is C. Individuals differ markedly in their clearance rates of individual drugs due to differences in absorption, blood volume, diseases of specific organs, variation in protein- and receptor-binding, other drugs present, and many undetermined factors. In the absence of specific knowledge regarding how the individual is clearing a specific drug at one time during treatment, the most reproducible and interpretable data will be obtained by measuring the trough level immediately before the next scheduled dose. (Tietz, pp. 843–851; Kaplan and Pesce, p. 977; Bishop et al, p. 533)

24. Measurement of urinary vanillylmandelic acid indicates the amount of hormone secreted by the

    A. Adrenal cortex
    B. Adrenal medulla
    C. Gonads
    D. Pituitary gland

The answer is B. Vanillylmandelic acid is the product of the common pathway of inactivated catecholamines, epinephrine, and norepinephrine. Epinephrine is the major product of the adrenal medulla, while most norepinephrine is produced by postganglionic sympathetic nerves. (Tietz, pp. 596–597; Kaplan and Pesce, p. 826; Bishop et al., pp. 328–329)

25. Urinary human chorionic gonadotropin (HCG) is used to detect

    A. Excessive estrogen secretion
    B. Fetal adrenal function
    C. Hypogonadism
    D. Pregnancy

The answer is D. HCG is produced by trophoblastic tissue, absorbed into the maternal plasma, and then excreted in the mother's urine. In a normal pregnancy, HCG rises in maternal blood soon after implantation of the fertilized ovum and doubles approximately every 2 days during the first trimester. A very slow decline then occurs through the rest of the gestation period. (Tietz, pp. 912–913; Kaplan and Pesce, p. 1147; Bishop et al., p. 335)

26. Elevated serum cortisol may indicate

    A. Addison's disease
    B. Cushing's syndrome
    C. Graves' disease
    D. Paget's disease

The answer is B. Cushing's syndrome is a group of symptoms caused by an excessive level of plasma cortisol due to overproduction by the adrenal cortex. Addison's disease is the result of inadequate secretion by the adrenal cortex; Graves' disease is a type of hyperthyroidism; and Paget's disease involves bone turnover. (Tietz, pp. 565–566; Kaplan and Pesce, p. 824; Bishop et al., p. 326)

27. Conjugation of bilirubin occurs primarily in the

    A. Common bile duct
    B. Hepatocytes
    C. Intestinal lumen
    D. Renal tubules

The answer is B. Bilirubin is formed in reticuloendothelial cells by the catabolism of heme and delivered via the plasma as a complex with albumin. Hepatocytes efficiently absorb this bilirubin, trap it intracellularly by protein-binding, conjugate it with glucuronic acid, and excrete it into the biliary tract. (Tietz, pp. 733–734; Kaplan and Pesce, pp. 648–650; Bishop et al., p. 439)

28. Urobilinogen is synthesized in

    A. Bone marrow
    B. Hepatocytes
    C. Intestinal lumen
    D. Kidney parenchyma

The answer is C. Hepatocytes excrete conjugated bilirubin into the bile duct for passage to the intestine. Intestinal bacteria degrade the molecule into derivatives which are collectively called urobilinogen. (Tietz, pp. 734–735; Kaplan and Pesce, p. 650; Bishop et al., p. 439)

29. Xanthochromic spinal fluid is an indicator of

    A. Bacterial meningitis
    B. Increased pressure of spinal fluid
    C. Increased protein concentration in spinal fluid
    D. Cerebral hemorrhage

The answer is D. Xanthochromia in spinal fluid is yellow pigmentation caused by the presence of bilirubin. The bilirubin results from breakdown of heme released from erythrocytes after bleeding into the brain or spinal column such as occurs in cerebral hemorrhage. (Kaplan and Pesce, p. 718)

30. The lecithin-sphingomyelin (L/S) ratio in amniotic fluid is used to indicate functional maturity of fetal

    A. Kidney
    B. Liver
    C. Lung
    D. Muscle

The answer is C. Increased synthesis of lecithin by fetal lungs begins in the 34th to 36th week of pregnancy. The alveolar lining becomes coated with this surface-active phospholipid which then appears in the amniotic fluid. An L/S ratio higher than 2.0 is associated with decreased risk of respiratory distress syndrome in the newborn period. (Tietz, pp. 921–923; Kaplan and Pesce, pp. 696–697; Bishop et al., pp. 486–487)

31. Samples for calcium analysis by atomic absorption spectrophotometry should be diluted with a lanthanum solution because lanthanum ions

   A. Blank for variations in flame temperature
   B. Blank for variations in lamp intensity
   C. Emit light used as the internal standard
   D. Enhance dissociation of calcium phosphate

The answer is D. Because of the requirement of a cool flame in atomic absorption spectrophotometry, some calcium salts are not broken into their component atoms; calcium phosphate is an example. The electrons in these anion-bound calcium atoms are then unable to absorb the incident wavelength of light and are not measured. Lanthanum binds the same anions more tightly than does calcium, which releases calcium from these salts. This allows the calcium electrons to achieve their ground state, absorb light energy, and be measured. (Tietz, p. 65; Kaplan and Pesce, p. 1053; Bishop et al., p. 274)

32. A fluorometer measures light that is

   A. Absorbed by excited electrons as they return to the ground state
   B. Emitted by excited electrons as they return to the ground state
   C. Polarized by the chemical reaction
   D. Scattered by insoluble particles produced by the reaction

The answer is B. The ground-state electrons of a fluorescent analyte absorb light of specific wavelengths, become excited for a few nanoseconds, and then re-emit their remaining energy as light of longer wavelengths. (Tietz, pp. 66–67; Kaplan and Pesce, p. 66; Bishop et al., p. 98)

33. When an ion-selective electrode interacts with its analyte, it produces a change in the electrode's

   A. Conductance
   B. Current
   C. Resistance
   D. Voltage

The answer is D. In an ion-selective electrode, ionic analyte reacts with an electrode surface producing a change in voltage at that surface. No current is allowed to flow. The analyte voltage is then compared to a known stable voltage and the meter expresses the difference between them as the concentration of analyte. (Tietz, p. 92; Kaplan and Pesce, 254; Bishop et al., p. 103)

34. Electrophoretic separation of proteins on cellulose acetate depends on the proteins differing in

    A. Concentration
    B. Molecular weight
    C. Net charge
    D. Number of peptide bonds

The answer is C. Electrophoresis is movement of an ion in an electric field. The rate of movement is directly proportional to the net charge of the ion. This principle is the basis for electrophoretic separation of serum proteins. The size of the ion also influences its mobility but this is not a major determinant when using cellulose acetate. (Tietz, 78; Kaplan and Pesce, p. 154; Bishop et al., p. 116)

35. In an automated instrument, the amount of carryover between consecutive samples *is not* affected by

    A. Rinsing the probe between samples
    B. Separating consecutive samples in a tubing by air segments
    C. Using a separate reaction chamber for each sample
    D. Using a serum blank

The answer is D. Carryover is the percent error produced by interaction or cross-contamination between adjacent samples. All techniques that rinse the components which touch adjacent samples or that increase the physical separation between adjacent samples decrease carryover. (Tietz, p. 166; Kaplan and Pesce, p. 264; Bishop et al., p. 126)

36. Chromatographic separation of a mixture of compounds depends on

    A. Some compounds being degraded by the mobile phase
    B. Some compounds being more strongly attracted to the stationary phase than others
    C. Some compounds being undetectable
    D. Some compounds being insoluble in the mobile phase

The answer is B. Chromatography separates solutes by competition between adsorption of solute to the support and dissolving it in the mobile phase. Thus compounds that differ in their attraction to the stationary phase can be separated from one another. (Tietz, pp. 105–106; Kaplan and Pesce, p. 76; Bishop et al., pp. 109–110)

37. In double-beam spectrophotometry, the beams referred to are

    A. Matched cuvettes
    B. Separate light paths

C. Supports for the instrument
D. The spectrum from a diffraction grating

The answer is B. The second (reference) light beam in a double-beam spectro-photometer continuously monitors the amount of light transmitted in the absence of sample chromogen. By expressing the absorbance of a sample as the ratio between its measuring light beam and the reference light beam, variation in lamp intensity or detector sensitivity are blanked. (Tietz, p. 51)

38. If serum protein electrophoresis is performed using higher voltage than the method calls for, which one of these *is least* likely?

A. Proteins migrate at a faster rate
B. Greater distance separates adjacent bands of protein
C. Less wick flow occurs
D. More heat is generated

The answer is C. Higher voltage causes increased heat production, which leads to drying of the support. Capillary action then draws buffer from the reservoirs onto the unsaturated support. This buffer movement is referred to as wick flow. The greater voltage also will cause the proteins to migrate faster and therefore separate more. (Tietz, p. 84)

39. The structure that carries urine from each kidney to the bladder is the

A. Collecting duct
B. Loop of Henle
C. Ureter
D. Urethra

The answer is C. Collecting ducts from each nephron empty urine into the ureter at the renal pelvis for transport to the bladder. (Tietz, p. 669; Kaplan and Pesce, p. 405; Bishop et al., p. 428; Graff, p. 3; Ross and Neely, p. 13)

40. Most of the solutes (e.g., amino acids, glucose, bicarbonate) that are filtered through the glomerulus are reabsorbed in the

A. Proximal convoluted tubule
B. Loop of Henle
C. Distal convoluted tubule
D. Collecting ducts

The answer is A. Over 80% of the volume of filtrate produced by each glomerulus is reabsorbed in the proximal convoluted tubule. A major fraction of most normally occurring solutes is reabsorbed in this volume. (Tietz, pp. 670–671; Kaplan and Pesce, p. 406; Bishop et al., 427; Graff, pp. 4–5; Ross and Neely, p. 16)

41. Which of these cells found in urinary sediment are characteristic of kidney disease and not just lower urinary tract disease?

    A. Erythrocytes
    B. Squamous epithelial cells
    C. Polymorphonuclear leukocytes
    D. Tubular epithelial cells

The answer is D. Blood cells may pathologically enter the urinary tract at any point. Squamous epithelium only occurs in the lower urinary tract. Renal tubular cells are only found in the upper urinary tract. (Kaplan and Pesce, p. 1016; Graff, pp. 107–108; Ross and Neely, p. 90)

42. Urinary sediment that contains red blood cells, red blood cell casts, and protein is characteristic of

    A. Acute glomerulonephritis
    B. Bladder infection
    C. Nephrotic syndrome
    D. Prostatic hypertrophy

The answer is A. In acute glomerulonephritis, breakdown of the basement membranes of glomeruli allows blood components, including erythrocytes and proteins, to enter the renal tubules. Subsequent concentration of the filtrate in the distal tubules results in formation of tubular casts which envelope the red blood cells present. (Kaplan and Pesce, p. 1021; Graff, p. 108; Ross and Neely, p. 21)

43. The dipstick that contains ferric ion produces a blue-green color on reaction with urine from a patient who has untreated

    A. Cystinuria
    B. Galactosemia
    C. Maple syrup urine disease
    D. Phenylketonuria

The answer is D. Phenylketones, which are excreted in high concentration in the urine of patients with untreated phenylketonuria, produce a blue-green chromogen with ferric ions in an acidic medium. (Graff, p. 249; Ross and Neely, p. 125)

44. In which of the glucose tolerances shown in the figure on p. 3 would you expect to find concurrent glycosuria?

    A. Curves 1 and 2
    B. Curves 1 and 3
    C. Curves 3 and 4
    D. Only curve 4

The answer is C. The normal renal threshold for glucose is a plasma level of 160 to 180 mg/dl. There is a limited amount of reabsorption mechanism in the proximal convoluted tubules. At blood glucose levels higher than the renal threshold the limited reabsorbtion allows excretion to the excess glucose in the urine. Both curves 3 and 4 exceed this renal threshold value. Individuals with renal disease, which includes many diabetic patients, may have even lower renal thresholds for glucose. (Tietz, p. 430; Kaplan and Pesce, p. 546; Bishop et al., p. 301; Graff, p. 36)

45. Hyaline casts are found in urinary sediment

    A. Following strenuous exercise
    B. From an alkaline urine
    C. Whenever an abnormal amount of protein is present
    D. When examined using bright light

The answer is A. Hyaline casts are not considered pathologic when they are the only abnormal finding following exercise. In these cases they are probably the result of temporary minor dehydration and consequent stagnation of renal filtrate. (Kaplan and Pesce, p. 1026; Graff, p. 108; Ross and Neely, p. 98)

46. Which of these sugars *cannot* be detected in urine using the copper reduction test?

    A. Fructose
    B. Galactose
    C. Lactose
    D. Sucrose

The answer is D. The copper reduction test detects carbohydrates by the reducing power of their free aldehyde groups. Sucrose has no free aldehyde group and does not produce the yellow-orange salts of oxidized copper. Sucrose is not absorbed or produced by the body. It only appears in urine as an artifact. (Kaplan and Pesce, pp. 1005–1006; Graff, p. 40; Ross and Neely, p. 82)

47. Bence Jones proteinuria may be detected by all *except*

    A. A dipstick for protein that uses the protein error of indicators
    B. Immunoelectrophoresis
    C. Precipitate formation with sulfosalicylic acid
    D. Precipitation between 40 and 60 °C

The answer is A. Bence Jones protein was originally recognized by its reversible precipitation between 40 and 60 °C. Sulfosalicylic acid is a general protein precipitant and will precipitate Bence Jones protein. Immunoelectrophoresis is the definitive method for identifying the specific types of immunoglobulin polypeptides (Bence Jones protein) that are being excreted. Bence Jones protein is not usually detectable using the dipstick method. (Kaplan and Pesce, p. 1005; Graff, p. 34)

48. Dipstick tests for urinary ketones use this substance to produce a purple chromogen.

    A. Diazotized sulfanilic acid
    B. p-Dimethylaminobenzaldehyde
    C. Sodium nitroferricyanide (nitroprusside)
    D. Sulfosalicylic acid

The answer is C. Sodium nitroferricyanide (nitroprusside) reacts with aceto-acetate in slightly alkaline conditions forming a purple chromogen. (Kaplan and Pesce, p. 1006; Graff, pp. 45–46; Ross and Neely, p. 77)

49. Calculate the creatinine clearance using these data obtained from a person with 1.73 m² body surface area:

    Serum creatinine: 1.8 mg/dl
    Urine creatinine: 54 mg/dl
    Urine volume: 640 ml/1440 min

    A. 3 ml/min
    B. 13 ml/min
    C. 21 ml/min
    D. 68 ml/min

The answer is B. The formula for calculating creatinine clearance is:

$$\frac{\text{urine concentration}}{\text{serum concentration}} \times \frac{\text{urine volume}}{\text{urine collection time}} \times \frac{1.73 \text{ m}^2}{\text{BSA}}$$

where urine and serum concentrations are both expressed in the same units, volume is milliliters, time is minutes, and BSA is body surface area in square meters. The calculated value has the units ml/min. (Tietz, p. 683; Kaplan and Pesce, p. 414; Bishop et al., p. 430)

50. Creatinine clearance is used to assess

    A. Hepatic blood flow
    B. Hepatic creatinine synthesis
    C. Renal plasma flow
    D. Renal glomerular filtration

The answer is D. Creatinine is filtered by glomeruli and excreted with little or no tubular reabsorption or secretion. Calculation of creatinine clearance essentially solves an equation for the amount of creatinine-containing plasma which must have been filtered in order to account for the amount of creatinine excreted in the urine. (Tietz, pp. 679–680; Kaplan and Pesce, p. 414; Bishop et al., p. 430)

CLS Review Questions

1. Criteria consistent with the diagnosis of diabetes mellitus include all *except*

   A. At least two serum glucose values of 200 mg/dl or more within 2 hr of an oral dose of glucose
   B. Fasting serum glucose of at least 140 mg/dl on more than one occasion
   C. Hypoglycemia within 3 hr of an oral dose of glucose
   D. Postprandial glycosuria in the absence of renal disease

The answer is C. NDDG criteria for the diagnosis of diabetes mellitus include either (1) a fasting serum glucose level greater than 140 mg/dl on more than one occasion or (2) two or more serum samples with glucose levels greater than 200 mg/dl following a meal. The latter values exceed the renal threshold for glucose and result in glycosuria. (Tietz, p. 433; Kaplan and Pesce, p. 544; Bishop et al., p. 304)

2. Hemoglobin A_{1c} is composed of

   A. 2,3-Diphosphoglycerate bound to hemoglobin
   B. Glucose covalently bound to hemoglobin
   C. The product of insulin action on glucose
   D. Two alpha chains and two delta chains

The answer is B. Hemoglobin A_{1c} is slowly produced by a nonenzymatic reaction during the life span of a circulating erythrocyte. It is the condensation product of glucose and the *N*-terminal amino group of beta-globin of hemoglobin. (Tietz, pp. 435–436; Kaplan and Pesce, p. 534; Bishop et al., p. 302)

3. Each of these enzymes may be used in methods for serum glucose measurement. Which one produces hydrogen peroxide when it reacts with glucose?

   A. G-6-PD
   B. Glucose oxidase
   C. Hexokinase
   D. Peroxidase

The answer is B. Glucose oxidase catalyzes the oxidation of glucose by molecular oxygen. The products are gluconic acid and hydrogen peroxide. There are several indicator reactions available for measuring the hydrogen peroxide. (Tietz, pp. 428–429; Kaplan and Pesce, p. 1033; Bishop et al., p. 299)

4. Cholesterol is removed from plasma by

   A. Apoprotein A
   B. Hepatic conjugation to bile acids
   C. Hepatic LDL receptors
   D. Lipoprotein lipases

The answer is C. Lipoprotein lipases remove triglycerides from triglyceride-rich VLDL and chylomicrons and successively produce IDL (intermediate-density lipoproteins) and then cholesterol-rich LDL particles. The apoliprotein B moiety in LDL binds to specific receptors in the liver, and the hepatocytes then internalize the particle and catabolize it. (Tietz, pp. 458–459; Kaplan and Pesce, p. 562; Bishop et al., p. 350)

5. The Friedewald formula for estimating LDL cholesterol is

LDL cholesterol = (total cholesterol) − (HDL cholesterol) − ⅕(total triglycerides)

This formula *should not* be used on serum with

A. HDL cholesterol higher than 40 mg/dl
B. Total cholesterol elevated for the age and sex of the patient
C. Triglyceride level higher than 400 mg/dl
D. No visible lipemia

The answer is C. The formula estimates cholesterol contained in LDL particles by subtracting cholesterol in other lipoprotein particles from total cholesterol. An essential assumption is that 20% (⅕) of VLDL particles is cholesterol and that measured triglyceride accurately estimates the amount of VLDL. When the triglyceride result is excessively high (>400 mg/dl) this assumption is not valid. (Tietz, p. 469; Kaplan and Pesce, p. 1212; Bishop et al., p. 356)

6. The serum protein electrophoresis pattern typical of nephrotic syndrome is

	Albumin	Alpha- and beta-globulins	gamma-globulins
A.	⇊	⇈	↓
B.	⇊	↓	⇈
C.	⇈	↓	Normal
D.	Normal	↑	⇊

The answer is A. In nephrotic syndrome, increased permeability of the glomerular membrane allows proteins of small molecular weight to escape into the urine in large quantities. Albumin and IgG, having relatively low molecular weights, are lost and the larger proteins, which remain in the plasma, appear to be present in increased concentration. (Tietz, pp. 318, 698–699; Kaplan and Pesce, p. 1314; Bishop et al., pp. 187–188)

7. Serum albumin may be quantitated by all of these methods *except*

A. Binding by bromcresol green
B. Electrophoresis at pH 8.6
C. Immunonephelometry
D. Sulfosalicylic acid precipitation

The answer is D. Bromcresol green, under appropriate conditions of pH and ionic strength, binds specifically to albumin. This shifts the wavelength of light absorbed by the dye. Electrophoresis of serum proteins results in a virtually pure band of albumin, in contrast to the other bands which are mixtures of proteins. Immunonephelometry is specific for an individual protein by virtue of antigen-antibody recognition. Sulfosalicylic acid is a general protein precipitant and is not specific for albumin. (Tietz, pp. 329–330; Kaplan and Pesce, p. 1269; Bishop et al., pp. 184–188)

8. Results of electrophoresis of proteins using a moderately hemolyzed serum show falsely increased

    A. Albumin
    B. Alpha$_1$-globulin
    C. Beta-globulin
    D. Gamma-globulin

The answer is C. Haptoglobin binds a small amount of hemoglobin in serum; the remaining free hemoglobin migrates electrophoretically with serum beta-globulins. (Tietz, p. 86; Bishop et al., p. 186)

9. Which serum isoenzyme *is least* likely to be elevated in a sample drawn 72 hr after an uncomplicated myocardial infarction?

    A. CK-MB (CK-2)
    B. CK-MM (CK-3)
    C. LD isoenzyme 1 (HHHH)
    D. Aspartate aminotransferase

The answer is A. After a myocardial infarction the MB isoenzyme of creatine kinase returns to the reference range earlier than any of the other enzymes listed, typically by the third day postinfarction. Preinfarction levels of CK-MM usually do not occur until the third or fourth day and aspartate aminotransferase returns to normal about 1 day later. LD isoenzyme 1 does not return to a normal level until 7 to 12 days following myocardial infarction. (Tietz, p. 384; Kaplan and Pesce, p. 501; Bishop et al., pp. 216, 218)

10. Which enzyme ratio is the best indicator of hepatitus?

    A. ALT/AST ratio
    B. Amylase/lipase ratio
    C. CK-MB/total CK ratio
    D. LD isoenzyme 1/LD isoenzyme 5 ratio

The answer is A. Hepatocytes are rich in both of these transaminases. The ratio of ALT to AST characteristically exceeds 1.0 in toxic or viral hepatitis. The other enzymes and isoenzymes listed are not found in significant quantities in hepatocytes. (Tietz, pp. 370–371; Kaplan and Pesce, p. 436; Bishop et al., p. 221)

11. Kinetic enzyme assay of a serum gives these data:

Time (min)	Absorbance
0	0.020
1	0.200
2	0.315
3	0.395
4	0.435
5	0.480

The best conclusion is

A. Readings are satisfactory; calculate the result.
B. Repeat the assay using diluted serum.
C. Calculate the result from the 0- to 3-min readings.
D. Calculate the result from the 3- to 5-min readings.

The answer is B. The rate of change of absorbance (change in absorbance per minute) is not constant for any of the data given. This indicates that there is insufficient substrate present for all of the enzyme molecules to be continuously active during the analysis, a condition referred to as substrate exhaustion. The rate of change of absorbance is therefore dependent on both enzyme concentration and substrate concentration. Use of less enzyme-containing serum will allow sufficient substrate for zero-order kinetics and still have a measurable change in absorbance. (Tietz, pp. 348–349; Kaplan and Pesce, pp. 938–939; Bishop et al., p. 212)

12. Significantly elevated serum amylase with normal urine amylase indicates

A. Acute pancreatitis
B. Chronic pancreatitis
C. Macroamylasemia
D. Salivary gland inflammation

The answer is C. Amylase is a sufficiently small protein to be filtered through normal renal glomeruli. This accounts for its rapidly increasing level in urine following a rise in serum value as is found in acute inflammation of the pancreatic or salivary glands. Macroamylasemia is a benign finding in which the small amount of amylase normally released into plasma is bound to an immunoglobulin, which results in a molecule too large for glomerular filtration. This enzyme-immunoglobulin complex is reactive in assays for amylase activity. Typical results are several times normal in serum but are not associated with any pathologic disorder. Chronic pancreatitis is not commonly associated with elevated amylase. (Tietz, p. 394; Kaplan and Pesce, p. 466; Bishop et al., p. 227)

13. Uric acid is the excretory form of nitrogen derived from

A. Amino acids
B. Creatinine

C. Purines
D. Urea

The answer is C. During degradation of purines (adenine and guanine), the ring structure is largely salvaged for reuse. That amount which escapes salvage is converted to uric acid and excreted into the urine. (Tietz, p. 684; Kaplan and Pesce, p. 410; Bishop et al., p. 417)

14. Urea can be measured by incubation with urease followed by all *except*

A. Formation of a colored product by reaction with diacetyl
B. Measurement of increased conductivity
C. Ion-selective electrode measurement of the ammonia produced
D. NADH consumption in a reaction catalyzed by glutamate dehydrogenase

The answer is A. Diacetyl condenses with urea in acid conditions producing a colored diazine. The urea molecule is broken down by urease into ammonium and carbonate ions. These ions increase the conductivity of the reaction mixture. Alternatively, the ammonium ions produced can be measured by an ion-selective electrode or by using them as substrate for glutamate dehydrogenase. (Tietz, pp. 677–678; Kaplan and Pesce, p. 1258; Bishop et al., p. 413)

15. Which one of these serum electrolyte results (mmol/L) *is most likely* in a serum with elevated lactate level?

	Na^+	K^+	Cl^-	CO_2 content
A.	125	4.5	100	10
B.	135	3.5	95	28
C.	145	4.0	90	15
D.	150	5.0	110	30

The answer is C. Excessive production of H^+ from lactic acid causes metabolic acidosis by depleting bicarbonate, the major component of CO_2 content. The total number of anions present is unchanged even though their relative amounts are abnormal. Therefore the concentrations of Na^+ and Cl^- do not become abnormal despite the increased anion gap. (Tietz, p. 657–659; Kaplan and Pesce, p. 1045; Bishop et al., pp. 285–286)

16. Neuromuscular irritability depends in part on the extracellular fluid concentration of

A. Complexed calcium
B. Ionized calcium
C. Protein-bound calcium
D. Total calcium

The answer is B. The functional form of calcium is the free ionized form. These functions include muscle contraction and neurotransmission as well as enzyme activation and its presence as a component of hydroxyapatite (the mineral deposit in bones and teeth). (Tietz, p. 705; Kaplan and Pesce, p. 491; Bishop et al., p. 274)

17. Which of these serum constituents has the largest effect on osmolality?

    A. Glucose
    B. Protein
    C. Sodium
    D. Urea

The answer is C. Osmolality is a measure of the molal activity of total solutes. In serum the molal concentration of sodium approximates its molar concentration and far exceeds that of any other serum solute. A glucose level of 100 mg/dl, e.g., is only 5.5 mmol/L, a urea nitrogen level of 15 mg/dl is only 2.5 mmol/L, and the molal concentration of 7 g/dl total proteins is very low due to the large molecular weights of proteins. (Tietz, pp. 666–667; Kaplan and Pesce, p. 234)

18. Calculate the blood pH from these arterial blood results.

    PCO$_2$:   45 mm Hg
    PO$_2$:   95 mm Hg
    Carbonic acid: 1.35 mmol/L
    Bicarbonate ion: 27 mmol/L
    CO$_2$ content: 28 mmol/L

    A. 6.62
    B. 7.40
    C. 7.51
    D. 7.62

The answer is B. Of the values given, only the bicarbonate and carbonic acid concentrations are needed to solve the Henderson-Hasselbalch equation for pH. The pK$_a$ for this buffer system is 6.1 in blood at 37 °C.

$$\text{pH} = 6.1 + \log \frac{HCO_3^-}{H_2CO_3}$$

(Tietz, p. 649; Kaplan and Pesce, pp. 396–398; Bishop et al., pp. 245, 255)

19. Compensation for acute metabolic acidosis is accomplished by

    A. Decreased rate of breathing
    B. Decreased reabsorbtion of renal bicarbonate
    C. Increased metabolic production of CO$_2$
    D. Hyperventilation

The answer is D. Low blood pH caused by metabolic acidosis stimulates respiration. This decreases the blood PCO$_2$ which shifts the ratio of bicarbonate to carbonic acid toward the normal, 20:1, and therefore shifts blood pH toward normal. At the same time, renal compensatory mechanisms conserve bicarbonate which also helps to restore the ratio of base to acid. (Tietz, p. 659; Kaplan and Pesce, p. 125; Bishop et al., p. 245)

20. Which of these conditions causes an increase in the P_{50} value of hemoglobin-oxygen dissociation?

    A. Decreased 2,3-diphosphoglcyerate (2,3-DPG)
    B. Elevated arterial pH
    C. Increased pCO_2
    D. Metabolic alkalosis

The answer is C. P_{50} is the amount of oxygen (mm Hg PO_2) required to convert 50% of hemoglobin to oxyhemoglobin. Increased P_{50} means that more oxygen is required, i.e., the hemoglobin-oxygen dissociation curve is shifted to the right. This shift occurs in acidosis (including increased PCO_2), fever, and increased level of erythrocyte 2,3-DPG. (Tietz, pp. 633–634; Kaplan and Pesce, pp. 394–395; Bishop et al., pp. 249–250)

21. Lead poisoning may be detected by elevated levels of all *except*

    A. Delta-aminolevulinate (ALA) dehydratase (porphobilinogen synthase) activity
    B. Free erythrocyte protoporphyrin
    C. 24-hr urinary lead
    D. Whole blood lead

The answer is A. Delta-ALA dehydratase (porphobilinogen synthase), an enzyme in the pathway of heme synthesis, is inhibited by lead. Lead also inhibits incorporation of iron into protoporphyrin IX, which results in accumulation of free protoporphyrin in erythrocytes. Whole blood is a good sample for detection of lead poisoning since lead tends to be sequestered and concentrated in erythrocytes. The small amount of excess lead that is free in plasma is excreted in the urine. (Tietz, p. 831; Kaplan and Pesce, p. 644; Bishop et al., p. 552)

22. Calculate the half-life of this drug in the circulation.

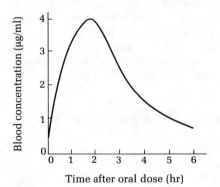

Time after oral dose (hr)

    A. ½ hr
    B. 1½ hr
    C. 2½ hr
    D. 4 hrs

The answer is B. The biologic half-life of a drug is the length of time required for any blood level to decay to half that level. In the diagram, the blood concentration is approximately 4 μg/ml at 2 hr and approximately 2 μg/ml at 3½ hrs; thus the level has dropped to one-half value in 3½ − 2 = 1½ hr. (Tietz, p. 846; Kaplan and Pesce, p. 965; Bishop et al., p. 527)

23. A patient with intermittent hypertension has an elevated value for urinary catecholamine metabolites (e.g., vanillylmandelic acid). This result may indicate

    A. Hyperaldosteronism
    B. Hypercortisolism
    C. Idiopathic hypertension
    D. Pheochromocytoma

The answer is D. Pheochromocytoma is an epinephrine-secreting tumor of the adrenal medulla. Epinephrine and norepinephrine have a chemical structure known as a catecholamine. They are both catabolized to vanillylmandelic acid, which is excreted in the urine. (Tietz, pp. 597–598; Kaplan and Pesce, p. 830; Bishop et al., p. 329)

24. Blood from a newborn has low thyroxine (T$_4$) and elevated thyroid-stimulating hormone (TSH) compared to reference ranges for that age. These results indicate

    A. Congenital hypopituitarism
    B. Congenital primary hypothyroidism
    C. Congenital secondary hypothyroidism
    D. Normal response to pregnancy-induced changes in maternal thyroid function

The answer is B. Production of T$_4$ by the thyroid gland has a negative feedback relationship with thyrotropin (TSH) produced by the anterior pituitary gland. Congenital abnormalities which prevent adequate production of T$_4$ result in a high level of TSH through this feedback loop. The elevated T$_4$ values seen in maternal serum are in artifact caused by estrogen-induced increase in synthesis of thyroxine-binding globulin. (Tietz, pp. 585–587; Kaplan and Pesce, p. 763; Bishop et al., p. 476)

25. Urinary HCG concentration is higher than nonpregnant values in all of these cases *except*

    A. Ten days following spontaneous abortion
    B. The 10th week of normal pregnancy
    C. Molar pregnancy (hydatidiform mole).
    D. Third trimester of normal pregnancy

The answer is A. HCG is produced by trophoblastic tissue, absorbed into the maternal plasma, and then excreted in the urine. Loss of trophoblastic tissue, such as happens in spontaneous abortion, results in rapid urinary clearance of the hormone resulting in values that are less than expected for the presumed period of gestation. Trophoblastic tumors, such as molar pregnancy, are associated with elevated values in the absence of pregnancy. In a normal pregnancy, HCG rises in maternal blood soon after implantation of the fertilized ovum and doubles approximately every 2 days during the first trimester. A very slow decline then occurs through the rest of the gestation period. (Tietz, pp. 912–913; Kaplan and Pesce, pp. 702–703; Bishop et al., p. 335)

26. A patient whose admission diagnosis is biliary obstruction has these laboratory results:

	Test	Result
Serum:	Conjugated bilirubin	Increased
	Total bilirubin	Increased
Urine:	Bilirubin	Positive
	Urobilinogen	Increased

Which result *is inconsistent* with the admission diagnosis?

A. Serum conjugated bilirubin
B. Serum total bilirubin
C. Urinary bilirubin
D. Urinary Urobilinogen

The answer is D. Urobilinogen is formed in the intestinal lumen by bacteria acting on excreted bile. A significant portion of the urobilinogen is then reabsorbed into the portal blood from which it is extracted and re-excreted on passage through the liver. Only the urobilinogen which escapes this hepatic removal reaches the kidneys for filtration into urine. A patient with obstructive liver disease would be expected to excrete less bilirubin into the intestine. Thus less urobilinogen would be formed, less would be reabsorbed, less would escape hepatic removal, and less would appear in the urine. Urinary bilirubin, on the other hand, is the water-soluble conjugated form. Regurgitation from canaliculi, caused by biliary obstruction, results in increased serum levels and filtration into urine. (Tietz, pp. 735–736; Kaplan and Pesce, p. 650; Bishop et al., p. 444)

27. When measuring serum bilirubin, the purpose of adding caffeine–sodium benzoate or methanol to the reaction mixture is to

A. Accelerate the reaction with conjugated bilirubin
B. Accelerate the reaction with unconjugated bilirubin
C. Destroy excess diazo reagent
D. Shift the wavelength absorbed by azobilirubin

The answer is B. Unconjugated bilirubin is poorly soluble in aqueous solution. It reacts very slowly with aqueous solution of the diazotizing color reagent unless an accelerating reagent, such as caffeine–sodium benzoate (Jendrassik-

Grof method) or methanol (Evelyn-Malloy method), is added. (Tietz, pp. 738–739; Kaplan and Pesce, p. 1234; Bishop et al., p. 442)

28. Which of these vitamins is absorbed poorly in pancreatic insufficiency?

    A. Vitamin A
    B. Vitamin B_1 (thiamine)
    C. Vitamin B_{12}
    D. Vitamin C

The answer is A. Vitamin A is a nonpolar derivative of isoprene and is poorly water-soluble. Without the assistance of pancreatic lipase and biliary bile acids, vitamin A is poorly soluble and therefore not efficiently absorbed from the intestine. (Tietz, p. 499; Kaplan et al., p. 475; Bishop et al., p. 368)

29. Amniotic fluid from an expectant mother in the 39th week of gestation gives these laboratory results:

    L/S ratio: 4.0
    Creatinine: 2.8 mg/dl
    Delta A_{450}:   0.008 (Liley zone I)

    These results indicate

    A. Inadequate fetal kidney function
    B. Intrauterine hemolysis
    C. Mature fetal lungs
    D. Small fetal body size

The answer is C. Increased synthesis of lecithin by fetal lungs begins in the 34th to 36th week of pregnancy. The alveolar lining becomes coated with this surface-active phospholipid which then appears in the amniotic fluid. An L/S ratio higher than 2.0 in amniotic flud is associated with maturation of the pulmonary lining and decreased risk of respiratory distress syndrome in the newborn period. Intrauterine hemolysis results in release of bilirubin, which absorbs light of 450-nm wavelength, into the amniotic fluid. Creatinine in amniotic fluid is a product of fetal muscle mass and correlates with fetal body weight. (Tietz, pp. 918–923; Kaplan and Pesce, 703, 705; Bishop et al., pp. 485–486)

30. When iontophoresis is used to collect sweat for chloride analysis, pilocarpine is used to

    A. Clean the skin area
    B. Complex with chloride
    C. Complete the circuit
    D. Induce sweat secretion

The answer is D. Pilocarpine is driven into the skin surface by iontophoresis (the migration of ions induced by direct current). It stimulates the production of sweat which is subsequently collected on preweighed filter paper or gauze for analysis of chloride or sodium. (Tietz, pp. 778–779; Kaplan and Pesce, p. 465; Bishop et al., p. 490)

31. These blood and spinal fluid samples were collected within 30 min of each other. Which of the pairs of glucose results indicates possible bacterial meningitis?

	Blood	Spinal fluid
A.	60 mg/dl	40 mg/dl
B.	100 mg/dl	60 mg/dl
C.	200 mg/dl	30 mg/dl
D.	200 mg/dl	120 mg/dl

The answer is C. In the absence of bacteria or increased numbers of leukocytes, the glucose concentration in spinal fluid should be 60 to 80% of the concurrent concentration in blood. (Tietz, p. 274; Kaplan and Pesce, pp. 722–723; Bishop et al., p. 489; Ross and Neely, p. 245)

32. A fuel-rich flame is used in atomic absorption spectrophotometry in order to

A. Avoid interference from other metals in the sample
B. Maximize production of oxide and hydroxide radicals
C. Minimize excitation of the analyte by heat
D. Prevent damage to the burner

The answer is C. A fuel-rich flame is cooler than an oxidant-rich flame. In order to absorb the incident wavelength of light efficiently, the electrons of the metallic analyte must be in their ground state. Excessive energy from a too-hot flame tends to excite some of these electrons and results in fewer ground-state electrons capable of light absorption. (Tietz, p. 63; Kaplan and Pesce, p. 64; Bishop et al., pp. 95–96)

33. Ion-selective electrodes compare the voltage of the measuring electrode to

A. A known stable reference voltage
B. The conductivity of the sample
C. The current required to establish the voltage
D. The resistivity of the sample

The answer is A. Potentiometric electrodes require two half-cells. One of them (the measuring electrode) produces a voltage which depends on the amount of the analyte being measured and the other (the reference electrode) is a source of known stable voltage. The meter then expresses the difference between these voltages which correlates with analyte concentration. (Tietz, pp. 87–88; Kaplan and Pesce, pp. 254; Bishop et al., p. 103)

34. In a radioactive competitive protein binding assay, the B_0 tube should read 30 to 70% of the total counts tube in order to

    A. Maximize specificity
    B. Maximize sensitivity
    C. Minimize the number of repeat analyses
    D. Minimize interference

The answer is B. The B_0 tube is the blank, i.e., standard of zero concentration. It determines the maximum amount of binding of labeled ligand when there is no competition from unlabeled ligand. If the labeled ligand is present in greater or lesser amount, the percent bound in the B_0 tube will change, the standard line will be shifted, and therefore the concentrations at which the method is most sensitive will shift. (Tietz, pp. 155–156; Kaplan and Pesce, p. 65; Bishop et al., p. 97)

35. Which of these characteristics is desired for a substance to be used as an internal standard?

    A. Does not change when instrument variables change
    B. Is more soluble in sample than the analyte is
    C. Is present in normal serum sample
    D. Produces a reaction detectable using the same type of detector as the analyte reaction

The answer is D. An internal standard is a substance added to all samples in constant concentration. The analyte and internal standard are then measured simultaneously, and any variation measured in the internal standard is assumed to have occurred also to the analyte. The measured signal from the internal standard is then used to correct the analyte signal to what it would have been had there been no variation. This correction assumes that the substance chosen for the internal standard reacts to all variables in the same way and to the same extent as the analyte. (Tietz, p. 63; Kaplan and Pesce, p. 65; Bishop et al., p. 97)

36. The PO_2 electrode measures

    A. H^+ generated by reaction at the electrode surface
    B. The amount of O_2 oxidized to hydrogen peroxide
    C. The number of electrons used to reduce O_2
    D. Voltage between the measuring half-cell and the reference half-cell

The answer is C. The PO_2 electrode differs from other commonly used electrodes in that it is amperometric instead of potentiometric. A known stable voltage is maintained between the anode and the platinum cathode. Oxygen diffuses through the membrane to the cathode where it is reduced by electrons furnished by the anode. The amount of current (electron flow) is measured and expressed as concentration of O_2. (Tietz, p. 98; Kaplan and Pesce, p. 257; Bishop et al., p. 252)

37. Thin-layer chromatography on silica gel uses solvent which is

    A. More polar than silica gel
    B. Less polar than silica gel
    C. More acidic than silica gel
    D. More basic than silica gel

The answer is B. Silica gel chromatography separates a mixture of solutes by differential competition between adsorption of each solute to the support and its solubility in the mobile phase. Since silica gel is polar, the solvent used with it is relatively nonpolar in order to maximize separation of the mixture. (Tietz, pp. 105–106; Kaplan and Pesce, p. 88; Bishop et al., p. 111)

38. Reactions in renal tubular cells which contribute to acid-base balance include all *except*

    A. Ammonia production from glutamine
    B. Bicarbonate production from the carbonic anhydrase reaction
    C. Exchange of Na^+ in tubular filtrate for H^+ in extracellular fluid
    D. Reabsorbtion of H_2O due to stimulation by antidiuretic hormone (ADH)

The answer is D. Renal tubular cells have an energy-requiring system which exchanges Na^+ in tubular filtrate for H^+ in body fluid. They also contain the enzyme glutaminase which splits ammonia from glutamine. The ammonia diffuses into filtrate and is converted to ammonium ion which cannot diffuse back. Renal tubular cells also contain carbonic anhydrase which accelerates the interconversion of carbonic acid with CO_2 and H_2O. This regulates the amount of bicarbonate available for excretion or reabsorption. ADH regulates reabsorption of water by the distal and collecting tubules. (Tietz, pp. 552, 654–656; Kaplan and Pesce, p. 409; Bishop et al., pp. 243–244; Graff, p. 6)

39. The ratio of serum urea nitrogen to serum creatinine is elevated by

    A. Decreased flow of renal tubular filtrate
    B. Decreased renal tubular reabsorbtion
    C. Increased blood pressure
    D. Increased hepatic blood flow

The answer is A. A significant amount of filtered urea is reabsorbed from renal tubules especially when the flow rate of the filtrate is decreased. Under the same conditions there is little or no change in the reabsorption of creatinine. This circumstance will cause less urea than creatinine to be cleared from the plasma. Thus the serum level will be elevated more than serum creatinine. (Tietz, pp. 676, 679; Kaplan and Pesce, p. 410; Bishop et al., p. 430)

40. The urine of a patient with light, clay-colored feces *is unlikely* to have

    A. Positive bilirubin
    B. Elevated urobilinogen
    C. Positive dipstick nitrite test
    D. Positive test for porphobilinogen

The answer is B. The normal color of stool is largely due to urobilins, the oxidation products of urobilinogens. Light clay-colored stools lack this pigmentation, often because of obstruction of the bile duct. This obstruction prevents entry of bilirubin glucuronide into the intestine and subsequent degradation of bilirubin into urobilinogens. The amount of urobilinogens reabsorbed into plasma is then decreased and this in turn decreases the amount filtered from plasma into the urine. (Tietz, p. 736; Kaplan and Pesce, p. 1007; Bishop et al., p. 444; Graff, p. 55; Ross and Neely, p. 80)

41. Approximately what percentage of nephrons are nonfunctional in a patient whose serum creatinine is 4 times normal?

    A. 10%
    B. 50%
    C. 85%
    D. 100%

The answer is C. At least half of the total nephrons are not required for homeostasis of renal excretion. This is demonstrated by the fact that renal transplant donors do not develop renal failure. Below that level, the serum creatinine level is approximately a linear function of the number of functional nephrons. (Tietz, p. 680; Kaplan and Pesce, p. 413; Bishop et al., p. 431)

42. The presence of granular casts in urinary sediment indicates any of these diseases except

    A. Cystitis
    B. Glomerular nephritis
    C. Pyelonephritis
    D. Renal failure

The answer is A. A cast is a mold of the renal tubule in which it has gelled. Cells that are trapped in the cast undergo degenerative changes producing granular casts. Cystitis is an infection of the lower urinary tract (e.g., the urinary bladder) and does not involve the kidney tubules. (Kaplan and Pesce, p. 1021; Graff, pp. 107–108; Ross and Neely, p. 97)

43. A urine sample which tests positive for ketones but negative for glucose is most likely from a patient who is suffering from

    A. Diabetes insipidus
    B. Diabetes mellitus
    C. Polydipsia
    D. Starvation

The answer is D. Ketones are the product of lipid catabolism producing acetoacetate in excess of the body's ability to catabolize it. This excessive lipid catabolism may occur in any state in which there is insufficient glucose metabolism for cellular energy requirements. (Tietz, p. 438; Kaplan and Pesce, p. 1006; Bishop et al., p. 297; Graff. p. 43; Ross and Neely, p. 77)

44. Which of these solutes contributes most to the osmolality of normal urine?

    A. Creatinine
    B. Phosphate
    C. Sodium
    D. Urea

The answer is D. Osmolality is a reflection of total dissolved solutes. Urine contains a far higher molar concentration of urea than any other solute. (Tietz, pp. 101, 967; Kaplan and Pesce, pp. 234, 1261)

45. These results are obtained on a sample for routine urinalysis:

    Appearance: cloudy, dark-colored
    Dipstick for hemoglobin: negative
    Microscopy: 25–50 RBCs per high-power field

    Plausible explanations of these results include all *except*

    A. The hemoglobin test may be falsely negative due to bleach.
    B. The hemoglobin test may be falsely negative due to ascorbic acid.
    C. The apparent RBCs may be truly yeast.
    D. The apparent RBCs may be truly WBCs.

The answer is A. Bleach is an oxidant which can cause the dipstick for hemoglobin to be artifactually positive. Ascorbic acid is a reducing substance which can cause it to be falsely negative. Even though the dipstick is less sensitive to intracellular hemoglobin than it is to free hemoglobin, it should detect this large amount of RBCs. The identification of the cells can be confirmed by addition of weak acetic acid which will lyse RBCs but not yeast or WBCs. (Graff, pp. 53–54, 74–76; Ross and Neely, p. 79)

46. Which of these crystals *is not found* in urinary sediment of an acidic urine?

    A. Cystine
    B. Calcium oxalate
    C. Triple phosphate
    D. Sodium urate

The answer is C. Triple phosphate is magnesium-ammonium phosphate, a salt that is poorly soluble at alkaline pH. At acid pH it dissociates into its soluble component ions. The other crystals listed are less soluble at acid pH than at alkaline pH. (Graff, pp. 84, 102; Ross and Neely, p. 100)

47. There are no dipstick tests for urinary ketones that measure

    A. Acetoacetic acid
    B. Acetone
    C. Diacetic acid
    D. Beta-hydroxybutyric acid

The answer is D. Acetoacetic acid and diacetic acid are synonyms. All dipsticks for ketones rely on reaction of acetoacetic acid with alkaline sodium nitro-prusside (nitroferricyanide) to produce a chromogen. Some also are able to detect acetone and some are not, but none detect beta-hydroxybutyric acid. (Graff, pp. 45–46; Ross and Neely, p. 77)

48. Creatinine clearance assesses the rate of

    A. Glomerular filtration
    B. Renal blood flow
    C. Renal tubular reabsorbtion
    D. Renal tubular secretion

The answer is A. Creatinine is filtered by glomeruli and then excreted with little or no tubular reabsorbtion or secretion. Calculation of creatinine clearance essentially is solving an equation for the amount of creatinine-containing plasma which must have been filtered in order to account for the amount of creatinine excreted in the urine. (Tietz, pp. 679–680; Kaplan and Pesce, p. 414; Bishop et al., p. 429)

49. Calculate the creatinine clearance using these data:

    Serum Creatinine: 1.8 mg/dl
    Urine creatinine: 54 mg/dl
    Urine volume: 640 mL/24 hr
    Body surface area: 1.25 m^2

    A. 1.1 ml/min
    B. 5 ml/min
    C. 13 ml/min
    D. 18 ml/min

The answer is D. The formula for calculation of creatinine clearance is:

$$\frac{urine\ concentration}{serum\ concentration} \times \frac{urine\ volume}{urine\ collection\ time} \times \frac{1.73\ m^2}{BSA}$$

where urine and serum concentrations are both expressed in the same units, volume is milliliters, time is minutes, and BSA is body surface area in square meters. The calculated value has the units ml/min. (Tietz, p. 683; Kaplan and Pesce, p. 414; Bishop et al., p. 430)

50. Which of these urine tests *does not* measure the concentrating ability of the kidney?

    A. Number of casts per low-power field
    B. Refractive index
    C. Osmolality
    D. Specific gravity

The answer is A. Refractive index, osmolality, and specific gravity are all influenced by the concentration of dissolved solutes in urine. On the other hand, casts are produced when Tamm-Horsfall protein congeals during stagnant flow of filtrate in renal tubules. (Graff, p. 107; Ross and Neely, pp. 71–74)

References

Bishop, M. L., Duben-Von Laufen, J. L., and Fody, E. P. (Eds.). *Clinical Chemistry Principles, Procedures, Correlations*, Philadelphia: Lippincott, 1985.

Graff, L. *A Handbook of Routine Urinalysis*, Philadelphia: Lippincott, 1983.

Kaplan, L. A., and Pesce, A. J. (Eds.). *Clinical Chemistry Theory, Analysis, and Correlation*, St. Louis: Mosby, 1984.

Ross, D. L., and Neely, A. E. *Textbook of Urinalysis and Body Fluids*, Norwalk, Conn.: Appleton-Century-Crofts, 1983.

Tietz, N. W. (Ed.). *Fundamentals of Clinical Chemistry* (2nd ed.). Philadelphia: Saunders, 1976.

Tietz, N. W. (Ed.). *Fundamentals of Clinical Chemistry* (3rd ed.). Philadelphia: Saunders, 1987.

Hematology | 2

Section Editor
Marian Schwabbauer, M.A.

Contributors
Robert Avery
R. Bamberg, Ph.D.
Joyce Behrens, M.S.
Jeannette R. Bell, M.S.
Barbara A. Brown
Linda L. Carr, M.S.
Bettye Covington, M.A.
Cheryl Dunlap-Katz
Mary Beth Englund
Valerie J. Evans
Dave Falleur, M.Ed.
Donald J. Gartner, M.S.
Wendy C. Goulder
Sue Holcomb
Lesline Jackson, M.S.
Jean Kaiser
Kathleen Kelly
John B. Kennedy, Ed.D.
Louann P. Lawrence, M.Ed.
Susan J. Leclair, M.S.
Karen G. Lofsness, M.S.
Natalie E. Lyter
Dorothy Mabary
Jayne Mathis
Mary Susan B. Osier
Kathleen M. Overton
Jan Parrish, M.Ed.
Terry Protextor
Roberta Ricker
Dorothy R. Schwartz
Sandra R. Sommer, M.S.
Anne Stiene-Martin, M.S.
Judith Sutherland, M.A.
Cheryl Swinehart, M.S.
Martha Thomas, M.S.
Karen Viskochil, M.S.
A. Ruth Winningham, M.S.
Jean Anne Zager Zorko, M.S.

CLT Review Questions

1. Coumarins are oral anticoagulants that

   A. Prolong the prothrombin time (PT)
   B. Act in the peripheral blood to decrease factor activity
   C. Have an immediate anticoagulant effect
   D. Are neutralized by protamine sulfate

The answer is A. The administration of coumarin interferes with the synthesis of factors II (prothrombin), VII, IX, and X in the liver and results in the production of antigenically active, yet biologically inactive, molecules of those factors. Coumarin produces its therapeutic effect within 36 to 48 hours. The PT is prolonged since it is sensitive to the presence of three of the four vitamin K–dependent factors: factors II, VII, and X. (Miale)

2. The following results were obtained for a patient.

Name of test	Results(sec)	Control (sec)
PT	25	12
Activated partial thromboplastin time (APTT)	80	32.5
Thrombin time	10	12

The APTT and PT are both corrected with normal serum, but not with adsorbed plasma. Select the factor deficiency that most likely is responsible for these results.

   A. I
   B. II
   C. V
   D. X

The answer is D. Once factor deficiency has been established and localized by screening tests, the specific deficiency can usually be identified by mixing experiments using normal barium sulfate–adsorbed plasma (containing fibrinogen and factors V, VIII, XI, and XII) and normal serum (containing factors IX, X, XI, and XII). Correction of both tests by serum, but not by adsorbed plasma, suggests a deficiency of factor X. (Henry)

3. A preoperative coagulation screening battery consists of a platelet count, PT, and APTT. An additional coagulation test that should be included in this battery is a

   A. Fibrinogen
   B. Factor VIII assay
   C. Bleeding time
   D. Fibrin split products

The answer is C. None of the three tests already in the battery evaluates platelet function. The bleeding time is dependent on functional platelets and capillary integrity and therefore is the most logical of the choices given to be included in the battery. (Harker)

4. Prothrombin is converted to thrombin by

    A. A complex of activated factors IX and VII, platelet factor 3, and calcium
    B. Calcium
    C. A complex of tissue factor, factor VII, and calcium
    D. A complex of activated factors X and V, platelet factor 3, and calcium

The answer is D. Prothrombin activation to form thrombin involves five components. It is well established that factor Xa serves as the protease that converts prothrombin to thrombin and that this reaction is greatly accelerated by three activator components: factor V, platelet factor 3 (phospholipid), and calcium (Ca^{2+}). (Wintrobe, p. 423)

5. Fibrinogen is converted to fibrin by

    A. Calcium
    B. Prothrombin
    C. Thrombin
    D. Thrombin in the presence of calcium

The answer is C. Thrombin is a proteolytic enzyme that acts directly on fibrinogen to form fibrin. (Miale, p. 840)

6. All of the following are true concerning the prothrombin group of plasma coagulation factors except

    A. Dependent on vitamin K for production
    B. Adsorbed by barium sulfate
    C. Normally present in serum, except for factor II
    D. Activated by thrombin

The answer is D. The prothrombin group (factors II, VII, IX, and X) are all dependent on vitamin K for their production. These factors are also adsorbed by barium sulfate; they are not activated by thrombin and, except for prothrombin, are not consumed during coagulation. (Brown, p. 182)

7. All of the following conditions cause an increased (prolonged) thrombin time except

    A. Hypofibrinogenemia
    B. Increased fibrin degradation products
    C. Heparin therapy
    D. Decreased prothrombin

The answer is D. Fibrin degradation products interfere with the polymerization of fibrin; heparin acts along with antithrombin III to neutralize thrombin; and decreased fibrinogen levels also result in prolonged thrombin times. However, the level of prothrombin has no effect on the thrombin time. (Henry)

8. Neither the PT nor the APTT detects a deficiency of

    A. Factor VIII
    B. Platelet factor 3
    C. Factor VII
    D. Factor IX

The answer is B. Phospholipid (platelet factor 3) is provided in the reagents used for both PT and APTT. Thus, a deficiency in platelet factor 3 would not be detected in either of these tests. (Harker)

9. The function of thromboplastin in the PT test is to

    A. Activate factor XII and provide platelet factor 3
    B. Provide tissue activator
    C. Activate factor VII and provide phospholipid
    D. Accelerate the reactions of factors VIII and V

The answer is C. When calcium and an excess of tissue extract, such as a saline extract of acetone-dried rabbit brain, are added to plasma, the factor VII present reacts with the tissue factor to form a reaction complex, which converts factor X to its active form, Xa. The Xa reacts with factor V, calcium, and the phospholipid in the thromboplastin to form extrinsic prothrombinase, which converts prothrombin to the proteolytic enzyme thrombin. Thrombin then reacts with fibrinogen to form fibrin. (Williams et al.)

10. Heparin inhibits the clotting of blood by neutralizing the effect of

    A. Calcium
    B. Platelets
    C. Thrombin
    D. Factor XIII

The answer is C. Heparin interacts with a lysine group on the antithrombin III molecule and exposes a reactive arginine group that, in turn, can inhibit the active serine group of thrombin. (Williams et al.)

11. Plasma is diluted in a fibrinogen activity determination to decrease the

    A. Amount of thrombin necessary
    B. Influence of inhibitors
    C. Amount of calcium needed
    D. Effect of deficiencies in other coagulation factors

The answer is B. Diluting the plasma in this procedure produces an excess of thrombin, thus nullifying the effect of inhibitors and making fibrinogen the rate-limiting factor. (Sirridge and Shannon)

12. The quality control data for normal and abnormal platelet controls have been acceptable for the last 6 days. A new lot number of normal control is run in parallel to the old lot number. What should be done with the following data?

	Results	Package Insert Acceptable Range
Old lot number	150.0×10^9/L	140.0×10^9/L $\pm$ 30.0×10^9/L
New lot number	160.0×10^9/L	200.0×10^9/L $\pm$ 30.0×10^9/L

A. Use the acceptable range of the old lot number.
B. Adjust the acceptable range to include the reading of 160.0×10^9/L.
C. Rerun the new lot number; then run a new vial of control, if necessary.
D. Recalibrate the instrument.

The answer is C. The instrument should not be recalibrated nor the acceptable range adjusted until the new lot number of control has been thoroughly evaluated by rerunning the new control on a new vial. If results are still out of range, check with the manufacturer for possible mislabeling of the control value. (Platt)

13. A male patient has a cancer with multiple metastases. His clotting studies include

PT:	11.8 sec
APTT:	31.2 sec
Factor V:	110%
Factor VIII:	200%
Platelet count:	550,000/μl

This patient most likely has

A. Vitamin K deficiency
B. von Willebrand's disease
C. Disseminated intravascular coagulation
D. No hemostatic problem

The answer is D. All of the values given fall within commonly accepted normal ranges; therefore, the patient most likely has no hemostatic problem. (Harker)

14. The following erythrocyte indices are obtained for a specimen:

MCV:	88 fl
MCH:	30 pg
MCHC:	34 g/dl

These erythrocytes on a Wright-stained smear should appear

A. Hypochromic: microcytic
B. Normochromic: microcytic
C. Normochromic: normocytic
D. Hypochromic: normocytic

The answer is C. The MCV, MCH, and MCHC are all within the normal range; therefore, the erythrocytes are normal-sized, with normal concentrations of hemoglobin. (Wintrobe)

15. An increase in metamyelocytes, myelocytes, and promyelocytes can be referred to as a(n)

A. Pelger-Huët anomaly
B. Shift to the left
C. Agranulocytosis
D. Leukocytosis

The answer is B. A shift to the left means there is an increase in immature granulocytes (metamyelocytes, myelocytes, promyelocytes, and blasts). Maturity of granulocytes is assessed by the shape of the nucleus, which changes from round to kidney bean to horseshoe to lobed. (Wintrobe)

16. The oscilloscope on a particle counter can give an indication of all of the following except

A. The variation in size of the particles being counted
B. A plug in the aperture or electric interference
C. Hemoglobin content of red cells
D. The number of particles present

The answer is C. The pulses as viewed on the oscilloscope are in proportion to the size and number of particles present in solution. A plug and electric line interference each has a characteristic electronic pattern on the oscilloscope. (Brown)

17. Automated, routine hematologic instruments have limitations that may result in significant errors in the

A. Hematocrit, due to inadequate erythrocyte lysis
B. Hemoglobin, if the lower threshold is not correctly set
C. MCH, due to incorrect MCV
D. Platelet count due to broken leukocytes

The answer is D. Erroneously high platelet counts can result from pieces of broken leukocytes being counted as platelets. The other three statements are false because hematocrit is measured on nonlysed erythrocytes; hemoglobin determination does not use a threshold setting; and MCH does not use MCV in its calculation. (Wintrobe, pp. 14, 17, 1052)

18. A tube is received in the laboratory containing only 2.0 ml of blood in an EDTA-anticoagulated vacuum tube designed for a 7.0-ml draw. Which of the following test results can be expected if this sample is used?

    A. Falsely lowered red cell count
    B. Falsely elevated hemoglobin
    C. Erroneously decreased microhematocrit
    D. Sedimentation rate (ESR) of expected value

The answer is C. Since excessive anticoagulant causes shrinkage of red cells, the ESR and microhematocrit are affected, whereas the number of red cells is not altered, nor is the amount of hemoglobin. Note that the calculated hematocrit as determined by Coulter counters does not reflect this morphologic change. (Brown, p. 8)

19. The following values were plotted during the first 6 days of a new lot of control for the leukocyte determination using an electronic particle counter:

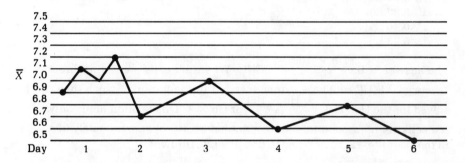

The coefficient of variation (CV) is 3.5%. Assume that these results are representative of the laboratory's usual performance on leukocyte counts in the normal and low ranges. Evaluation of the statistical pattern and the coefficient of variation indicates that

    A. Corrective action is unnecessary since the CV and plotted data are acceptable.
    B. A dilutor check is necessary.
    C. The control may be deteriorating.
    D. Calculation of a new mean and standard deviation is necessary.

The answer is C. Continuously increasing variance in one direction points to a segment, control sample, or instrument problem. If the drift were upward, one would first suspect a dilutor error. In this instance, the drift is downward; therefore, the most likely factor is a deterioration of the control. Other possibilities are reagent deterioration and an electronic problem with the counting instrument. (Brown)

20. What action would you take if, while performing a differential count on a capillary blood smear, you observed no platelets?

   A. Report the finding to your supervisor immediately.
   B. Request a venous sample for an absolute platelet count.
   C. Look at the edge of the smear for platelet clumping.
   D. Report out the absence of platelets.

The answer is C. Because of the nature of platelets, slides not prepared immediately after a capillary puncture may have excessive platelet clumping along the tail and margins of the stained slide. Slides with excessive clumping cannot be properly evaluated for platelet numbers and should be remade. (Brown)

21. A patient's hemoglobin level is 12.3 g/dl. The erythrocytes appear normochromic on the Wright-stained smear. The hematocrit value that correlates with these data is

   A. 0.34 L/L
   B. 0.37 L/L
   C. 0.40 L/L
   D. 0.43 L/L

The answer is B. $\dfrac{Hb \times 100}{Hct} = MCHC$. When red cells are normochromic, an "average" MCHC of 33.3% can be inserted in the formula, which then can be solved for the Hct. Hct $= \dfrac{Hb \times 100}{33.3}$ or Hb $\times$ 3. This relation holds only if the red cells are normochromic (have a normal MCHC of approximately 33–34%). In the example, 12.3 $\times$ 3 = 36.9% or 0.369 L/L. (Brown)

22. A falsely elevated hematocrit is obtained on a defective centrifuge. Which of the following values will *not* be affected?

   A. MCH
   B. MCV
   C. MCHC
   D. All of the above

The answer is A. Both the MCV and the MCHC use the hematocrit in their calculation. Therefore, only the MCH would be unaffected by a falsely elevated hematocrit. (Henry)

23. A patient's hematologic results are as follows:

WBC: 2.0×10^9/L
RBC: 3.83×10^{12}/L
Hb: 11.5 g/dl
Hct: 340 L/L
Plt: 60.0×10^9/L

Blood smear evaulation for quality control purposes reveals acceptable cell distribution; normocytic-normochromic red cells; eight leukocytes per 10 × field; 10 platelets per oil-immersion field. The next step is to

A. Report the results as obtained.
B. Repeat the leukocyte count.
C. Repeat the platelet count.
D. Repeat the red cell indices.

The answer is C. In general, one platelet per oil-immersion field is equal to 10,000 to 40,000 per microliter ($10-40 \times 10^9$/L). Therefore, this patient's platelet count would be expected to be greater than 100×10^9/L and should be repeated. All the other data given are compatible. (Platt)

24. Using the estimated mean and standard deviation from the previous month, the following results were obtained the first 2 days new controls were used:

Instrument: particle counter
Dilutor: automatic
Assay values(published)
    Normal WBC: 8.2 ± 0.6
    Abnormal WBC: 15.5 ± 0.9
    Normal RBC: 4.58 ± 0.09
    Abnormal RBC: 1.54 ± 0.12

Laboratory Values

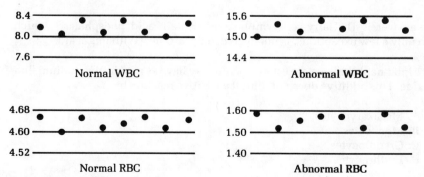

A possible source of error is

A. Poor mixing of controls
B. No obvious error indicated
C. Lysing agent expired
D. Diluent contaminated with bacteria

The answer is B. Standard quality control limits are ±2 SDs. Since all the results fall within the accepted published range, no obvious error is present. No trends are represented in the data. Poor mixing would produce data that had a trend, and expired lysing reagent would tend to increase the WBC determinations. Diluent contamination would affect both WBC and RBC determinations, with an upward trend as bacterial growth increased. (Henry)

25. In a typical instance of iron deficiency anemia, all the following would be present *except*

A. Microcytes, hypochromia, poikilocytes
B. Small platelets and an elevated platelet count
C. Decreased serum iron
D. Decreased total iron-binding capacity (TIBC)

The answer is D. The characteristic morphologic picture of iron deficiency anemia is hypochromic and microcytic. Usually the iron is decreased, and the TIBC is increased. Another finding often overlooked is that platelets are often smaller and increased in number. (Williams et al.)

26. Cells that demonstrate a positive reaction with the tartrate-resistant acid phosphatase stain include lymphocytes of

A. T cell acute lymphocytic leukemia
B. Infectious lymphocytosis
C. Non-T, non-B Tdt-positive acute lymphocytic leukemia
D. Hairy-cell leukemia

The answer is D. Hairy-cell lymphocytes contain acid phosphatase, which, with only a few exceptions, is not degraded by tartrate. (Williams et al.)

27. Alpha-naphthol-acetate esterase stain may have as an additive sodium fluoride. This additive does *not* inhibit a positive reaction by

A. Megakaryocytes
B. Monocytes
C. Granulocytes
D. Erythrocytes

The answer is C. Positivity in granulocytes is not affected by the addition of sodium fluoride as it is in monocytes. (Williams et al.)

28. Lymphoblasts in acute lymphocytic leukemia would most likely show a positive staining reaction with

   A. PAS (periodic acid-Schiff)
   B. Sudan black B
   C. Myeloperoxidase
   D. Nonspecific esterase

The answer is A. In most instances of acute lymphocytic leukemia, at least some of the lymphoblasts stain positively with the PAS stain. The other stains listed usually stain positively with cells of the granulocytic, and sometimes monocytic, cell lines, but usually do not stain lymphoblasts. (Miale)

29. To calculate the leukocyte alkaline phosphatase score on a blood smear

   A. Add the scores for the 100 neutrophils counted
   B. Average the scores for all cells counted
   C. Add the scores for the 100 leukocytes counted
   D. Calculate the percentage of positive-reacting cells

The answer is A. One hundred mature neutrophils in a thin area of the smear are scored 0 to 4 according to the staining characteristics. Adding these scores gives the total leukocyte alkaline phosphatase activity. Increased activity is seen in infections with leukocytosis (a leukemoid reaction), and decreased activity is seen in chronic granulocytic leukemia. The reference values are approximately 20 to 100. (Henry)

30. Which one of the following sets of hematologic results would be within the reference interval (normal values) for a 25-year-old woman?

	Hb (g/dl)	Hct (L/L)	RBC Count $\times 10^{12}/L$	WBC Count $\times 10^4/L$	Plt Count $\times 10^9/L$
A.	11.6	.34	4.2	6.2	390
B.	13.8	.40	4.6	10.1	300
C.	14.3	.45	5.9	7.5	125
D.	15.7	.48	5.3	3.6	275

The answer is B. Only those values given in option B all fall within the commonly accepted reference values. In C, the platelet count is low; in A, the hemoglobin is low: and in D, the white cell count is low. (Henry)

31. What affect would the use of a buffer with a pH of 6.0 have on a Wright-stained smear?

   A. Red cells would be too pink.
   B. White cells would be well differentiated.
   C. Red cells would be too blue.
   D. Red cells would lyse.

The answer is A. The pH of the buffer is critical in a Romanowsky stain. When the pH is too low (usual range is 6.4–6.7), the red cells take up more of the acid dye (eosin) and become too pink, whereas the white cells do not differentiate well, giving poor nuclear detail. (Brown)

32. Which of the following red cell inclusions can be detected with a supravital preparation that uses new methylene blue N as the dye reagent, but is not visible with Romanowsky staining?

    A. Howell-Jolly bodies
    B. Heinz bodies
    C. Ribosomal RNA (reticulum)
    D. Siderotic granules

The answer is B. There are only a few red cell inclusions that cannot be seen on a Romanowsky stain. Heinz bodies, since they are composed of precipitated globin, have the same net charges as nonprecipitated globin and therefore are not perceptible with a stain based on acid-base principles, such as the Romanowsky stains. (Brown)

33. High leukocyte alkaline phosphatase activity is least characteristic of

    A. Acute lymphoblastic leukemia
    B. Chronic myelogenous leukemia
    C. Leukemoid reaction
    D. Polycythemia vera

The answer is B. Leukocyte alkaline phosphatase activity reflects intracellular metabolic activity. Using the method of Kaplow, the score is high in leukemoid reactions and leukocytosis due to infection. It is also high in pregnancy and in newborns. Low values are found in acute and chronic myelogenous leukemias, monocytic leukemias, and paroxysmal nocturnal hemoglobinuria. (Henry)

34. Which of the following contain RNA and are usually identified by staining with brilliant cresyl blue or new methylene blue?

    A. Heinz bodies
    B. Reticulocytes
    C. Siderocytes (Pappenheimer bodies)
    D. Howell-Jolly bodies

The answer is B. Brilliant cresyl blue and new methylene blue precipitate erythrocyte ribosomes into a network so that reticulocytes can be distinguished from cells containing Heinz bodies, Pappenheimer bodies, or Howell-Jolly bodies. (Wintrobe)

35. If on a manual white count you count 36 cells in all nine square millimeters on a Neubauer-ruled hemacytometer with a 1:10 dilution, what is the patient's total WBC count?

A. $0.4 \times 10^9/L$
B. $2.5 \times 10^9/L$
C. $4.0 \times 10^9/L$
D. $8.0 \times 10^9/L$

The answer is A.

$$\frac{\text{Number of cells counted}}{\text{Volume counted}} \times \text{dilution} = \text{Number of cells per cubic millimeter}$$

$$\frac{36}{0.9} \times 10 = 400/mm^3, \text{ or } 0.4 \times 10^9/L$$

(Brown)

36. Calculate the hemoglobin concentration of the unknown.

   Hb standard: assay 72 mg/dl
   Dilution: 0.02 ml blood added to 5.0 ml diluent
   Absorbance readings: standard: 0.47
                           unknown: 0.35

   A. 5.4 g/L
   B. 11.0 g/dl
   C. 13.6 g/dl
   D. 24.0 g/dl

The answer is C.

72 mg/dl = 0.072 g/dl

0.02 ml blood + 5.0 ml diluent = 1:251 dilution

$$\frac{\text{Absorbance of unknown}}{\text{Absorbance of standard}} = \frac{\text{value of diluted unknown}}{\text{value of standard}}$$

$$\frac{0.35}{0.47} = \frac{\text{value of unknown}}{0.072 \text{ g/dl}} = 0.054 \text{ g/dl} \times 251 = 13.55 \text{ g/dl}$$

(Henry)

37. The leukocyte count for a patient is $28.0 \times 10^9/L$. The differential shows 58 metarubricytes (orthochromatic normoblasts) and 10 rubricytes (polychromatophilic normoblasts) per 100 leukocytes. The leukocyte count is closest to

   A. $2.8 \times 10^9/L$
   B. $16.7 \times 10^9/L$
   C. $17.7 \times 10^9/L$
   D. $28.0 \times 10^9/L$

The answer is B. The nucleated erythrocytes are counted as leukocytes; thus, the leukocyte count must be corrected using the following formula:

$$\frac{\text{Uncorrected WBC} \times 100}{100 + \text{nucleated RBC}} = \text{corrected WBC}$$

$$\frac{28.0 \times 10^9 \times 100}{100 + 58 + 10} = \frac{2800 \times 10^9}{168} = 16.7 \times 10^9/\text{L}$$

(Henry)

38. In an adult male, the approximate plasmacrit of circulating whole blood is

    A. .35 L/L
    B. .45 L/L
    C. .55 L/L
    D. .65 L/L

The answer is C. The plasmacrit is the volume of plasma, and the hematocrit the volume of red cells occupying a given volume of blood. The normal hematocrit for an adult male is .43 to .47 L/L. Therefore, the plasmacrit is approximately .55 (1.00 − .45) L/L. (Miale)

39. An osmotic fragility test is performed on blood incubated 24 hr at 37 C.

    The results are as follows:

% NaCl	%Hemolysis
0.80	0
0.75	3
0.70	19
0.65	48
0.60	79
0.55	100

From these data you can conclude that the patient has

    A. Spherocytosis
    B. Sickle cells
    C. Codocytes
    D. Normal red cells

The answer is A. These cells show complete lysis in a far more concentrated saline solution than normal red cells would, indicating that they are spherical, and thus osmotically fragile. (Henry)

40. The leukocyte count for an adult patient is 18 × 10⁹/L. The differential shows:

Segmented neutrophils:	56%
Band neutrophils:	5%
Lymphocytes:	25%
Monocytes:	10%
Eosinophils:	3%
Basophils:	1%

The above data reveal an absolute increase in

A. Segmented neutrophils and eosinophils
B. Lymphocytes and monocytes
C. Monocytes and segmented neutrophils
D. Eosinophils and lymphocytes

The answer is C. Although the percentages for segmented neutrophils and monocytes fall within the normal range, these forms are increased in absolute numbers because the total count is increased. (Henry)

41. Below are hematologic anticoagulants and corresponding characteristics of each. Select the one anticoagulant that does not match its characteristic.

A. Dipotassium EDTA—prevents platelet clumping
B. Sodium citrate—used for routine coagulation studies
C. Heparin—suitable for blood smears
D. Double oxalate—produces morphologic artifacts

The answer is C. Heparin is not suitable for blood smears because it gives a bluish background on Romanowsky-stained smears. (Brown)

42. A student consistently makes peripheral blood smears that are too thin. You instruct him or her to try

A. Using a smaller drop of blood
B. Using only capillary blood
C. Increasing the angle of the spreader slide
D. Applying more pressure on the spreader slide

The answer is C. Decreasing the angle of the spreader slide results in an even thinner preparation, whereas increasing the angle should result in a smear of correct thickness. Using a smaller drop of blood or applying more pressure can result in a thinner smear. Both capillary and anticoagulated blood should render equally satisfactory smears if other factors are correct, such as angle and size of blood drop. (Brown)

43. The development and production of basophils occurs primarily in the

A. Lymphatic system
B. Spleen
C. Liver
D. bone marrow

The answer is D. Granulocytes develop in the bone marrow from myeloblasts. Basophils are granulocytes and also mature from this cell line. (Williams et al.)

44. The most reliable criterion used to determine the maturity of a Wright-stained blood cell is the

A. Size of the nucleus
B. Color of the nucleus
C. Nucleus-to-cytoplasm ratio
D. Structure of the nuclear chromatin

The answer is D. The maturation stage of blood cell can best be determined by evaluation of the nuclear chromatin structure or pattern. The chromatin pattern changes are more consistent. Size or color variables can be affected by slide preparation, quality of stain, and/or staining techniques. (Diggs, p.3)

45. Which characteristic differentiates the myelocyte from the other cells in myelocytic maturation?

A. A kidney bean–shaped nucleus
B. Coarse nuclear chromatin
C. Presence of nucleoli
D. Appearance of specific granules

The answer is D. It is sometimes difficult to identify the early myelocyte. Identification depends on noting the first appearance of specific granules. Other morphologic features that are helpful include the fine texture of the nuclear chromatin, absence of nucleoli, and lack of indentation in the nucleus. (Henry)

46. Hematologic testing on an adult patient provides the following data:

Hb: 7.5 g/dl
Hct: .26 L/L
WBC: 14.6 × 10⁹/L
Neutrophils: 80%
Lymphocytes: 17%
Monocytes: 3%

These results would best correlate with

A. Normochromic RBCs; relative lymphocytopenia
B. Hypochromic RBCs; absolute lymphocytopenia
C. Normochromic RBCs; absolute lymphocytopenia
D. Hypochromic RBCs; relative lymphocytopenia

The answer is D. The MCHC is 28.9%, which is below normal (normal = 32–35%), indicating hypochromia. To determine whether the lymphocytopenia is absolute or relative, one must determine the actual number of lymphocytes per liter. Thus, 17% of 14.6 × 10⁹/L is 2.5 × 10⁹ lymphocytes per liter. The normal adult lymphocyte count is 1.5 to 4.5 × 10⁹/L. (Wintrobe)

47. A reactive lymphocyte, such as those seen in infectious mononucleosis, differs morphologically from a normal lymphocyte in that it often

    A. Contains nucleoli
    B. Is smaller
    C. Has less cytoplasm
    D. Is regularly shaped

The answer is A. The reactive (or atypical) lymphocytes seen in infectious mononucleosis are usually larger than normal, with irregular margins and peripheral basophilia. They often appear immature, with an open chromatin pattern and nucleoli. (Brown)

48. Which of the following is *not* a characteristic of a monocyte?

    A. Large cell, 14 to 20 μm in diameter
    B. Bright blue cytoplasm
    C. Vacuoles in cytoplasm
    D. Folded nucleus with lacy chromatin pattern

The answer is B. The classic description of a monocyte is a large cell with abundant, blue-gray cytoplasm containing many fine azurophilic granules. The nucleus can be round, kidney-shaped, or lobulated, with a fine, basket-weave chromatin pattern. The nucleus may be folded, and the cytoplasm may contain vacuoles. (Brown)

49. Inclusions that may be observed within leukocytes are

    A. Howell-Jolly bodies
    B. Basophilic stippling
    C. Malarial parasites
    D. Döhle bodies

The answer is D. Howell-Jolly bodies are small, round, basophilic inclusions that represent nuclear remnants in the red cell. Basophilic stippling refers to punctate basophilic inclusions in the red cell. Malarial parasites can be seen in the red cells of patients suffering from malaria. (Williams et al.)

50. The majority of electronic cell counters used in small and medium-sized hematology laboratories count cells based on

    A. The impedance principle
    B. Light scattering
    C. Light absorption
    D. Reverse dark field

The answer is A. Examples of cell counters that are widely used in small and medium-sized hematology laboratories and that use the impedance principle (also known as electric conductivity or electrolyte displacement) are instruments produced by Coulter and J. T. Baker. The light scattering (or reverse dark field) principle is used in instruments produced by Technicon and Ortho. (Lee)

CLS Review Questions

1. The patient's plasma has a normal prothrombin time (PT) and an activated partial thromboplastin time (APTT) of 164 sec. The APTT is not corrected by factor VIII–deficient plasma but is corrected by factor IX–deficient plasma. Which factor appears to be deficient?

   A. VIII
   B. IX
   C. Either XI or XII
   D. None

The answer is A. Since the PT is normal, one can assume that the extrinsic system and common pathway factors are functioning normally. This leaves factor VIII, IX, XI, or XII as possibly deficient. Since the APTT is corrected by factor IX–deficient plasma, factor IX must be present in the patient's plasma. When factor VIII–deficient plasma does not correct the APTT, the patient's plasma is presumed to lack normal factor VIII activity. (Miale)

2. A preoperative patient with a history of frequent bleeding episodes has a normal PT but an abnormal (135 sec) APTT, which is corrected by the addition of each of the following: normal plasma, factor VIII–deficient plasma, and factor IX–deficient plasma. Which factor assay(s) should be run?

   A. VIII
   B. IX
   C. XI and XII
   D. None; there is an antibody present

The answer is C. Correction with normal plasma rules out the presence of an antibody. Correction with VIII–deficient and IX–deficient plasma rules out factor VIII and IX deficiencies. Therefore, the factors left as possibilities are XI and XII. (Miale)

3. Each of the following drugs enhances the effect of oral anticoagulants (vitamin K antagonists), *except*

   A. Barbiturates
   B. Indomethacin
   C. Phenylbutazone
   D. Clofibrate

The answer is A. A number of drugs may either potentiate or inhibit the hypoprothrombinemic effect of oral anticoagulants. Indomethacin, phenyl-butazone, and clofibrate potentiate the effect of coumarin. These drugs act by displacement of the albumin-bound drug, thus increasing the concentration of free drug available for inhibition of vitamin K. Barbiturates reduce the effect of the oral anticoagulants by causing increased metabolism and more rapid clearance. (Harker)

4. A patient with dysfibrinogenemia will have a normal

   A. Immunologic fibrinogen level
   B. Thrombin time
   C. APTT
   D. Kinetic fibrinogen level

The answer is A. In most dysfibrinogenemias, the fibrinogen does not polymerize properly. Therefore, tests based on fibrin formation, such as the thrombin time, APTT, and kinetic fibrinogen assay show abnormal results, whereas immunologic and precipitation methods show normal levels. (Williams et al.)

5. Laboratory findings in acute disseminated intravascular coagulation (DIC) reflect abnormalities in which of the following phases or stages of blood coagulation?

   A. Phase 1 (platelet activation)
   B. Phases 1 and 2 (thromboplastinogenesis)
   C. Phases 1, 2, and 3 (thrombogenesis)
   D. Phases 1, 2, 3, and 4 (fibrin formation and fibrinolysis)

The answer is D. In DIC, either the intrinsic or extrinsic system or both are activated, resulting in the deposition of fibrin and increased fibrinolysis. Laboratory findings reflect the total involvement of the coagulation mechanism. (Miale)

6. A patient has a PT of 30 sec (control 11.2 sec). Vitamin K is administered IV; 24 hr later, the patient's PT is 17 sec. These findings are suggestive of

   A. Liver disease
   B. Factor V deficiency
   C. Obstructive jaundice
   D. Congenital factor VII deficiency

The answer is C. In liver disease administration of vitamin K does not correct the PT since the diseased liver cannot utilize vitamin K. Administration of vitamin K does not raise the level of factors in congenital factor deficiencies. If vitamin K is given parenterally, however, the PT is corrected in obstructive jaundice since the defective absorption mechanism in the liver is bypassed. (Miale)

7. A platelet aggregometer is basically a

    A. Densitometer
    B. Nephelometer
    C. Fluorometer
    D. Photometer

The answer is B. In the platelet aggregation test, the change in turbidity of platelet-rich plasma is measured after the addition of various aggregating agents. Since a nephelometer is used to detect the change in turbidity, the aggregometer is more closely related to this instrument than to the others. (Henry)

8. The cause of a *false* positive result in an immunologic fibrin degradation products test could be a(n)

    A. Inadequately clotted specimen
    B. One-hour delay in performance of the test
    C. Abruptio placentae
    D. Pulmonary embolism

The answer is A. An inadequately clotted specimen will give a *false* positive result in those test systems using an antifibrinogen antibody. Patients with abruptio placentae or pulmonary embolism often have elevated fibrin degradation products as a result of intravascular coagulation (true positive). (Sirridge and Shannon)

9. A decreased anticoagulant response to heparin therapy may be caused by decreased levels of

    A. Antithrombin III
    B. Platelet factor 4
    C. Factor XIII
    D. Endothelial component thromboxane

The answer is A. Antithrombin III acts (with heparin as a catalyst) to neutralize factors Xa, XIa, IXa, thrombin, and plasmin. Therefore, low levels of antithrombin III result in decreased neutralization of these factors in the face of high levels of heparin, since heparin only acts as a catalyst. (Harker)

10. The following results are obtained on a specimen from a 60-year-old woman:

    PT: 21.9 sec (normal: 11.5–15.0 sec)
    APTT: 70.2 sec (normal: 35–45 sec)
    Thrombin time: 120 sec (normal: 13.0–20.0 sec)
    Thrombin time dilution (1:4): 40.0 sec (1 part patient's plasma plus 3 parts normal plasma)

These findings are more consistent with

A. DIC
B. Heparin therapy
C. Hypofibrinogenemia
D. Lupus inhibitor

The answer is B. Prolonged values that do not correct with the addition of normal plasma are due to either an inhibitor or an anticoagulant. In this instance, with all three tests prolonged, the most likely explanation is heparin therapy. A lupus inhibitor does not prolong the thrombin time. (Henry)

11. The protamine sulfate in the protamine sulfate paracoagulation test

A. Aggregates platelets
B. Polymerizes fibrinogen to form a clot
C. Precipitates fibrin monomer complexes
D. Neutralizes heparin

The answer is C. Addition of weak protamine sulfate to plasma-containing fibrin monomer causes precipitation of soluble fibrin monomer/fibrinogen/ fibrin degradation product complexes. (Williams et al.)

12. The platelet aggregation curve below shows aggregation as follows:

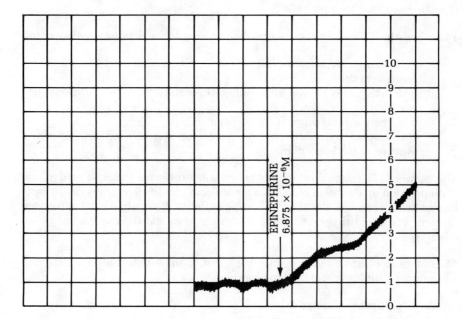

	Primary	Secondary
A.	Yes	No
B.	No	Yes
C.	Yes	Yes
D.	No	No

The answer is C. This normal curve shows a primary phase of aggregation just after the addition of 6.875×10^{-6}M epinephrine, followed by a secondary response caused by the release of endogenous ADP during the initial phase of aggregation. (Henry)

13. If normal aged serum and normal alumimum hydroxide–adsorbed citrated plasma are mixed in a test tube, and an APTT is performed on this mixture, which factor is still needed to form a normal clot?

    A. Factor V
    B. Factor VIII
    C. Fibrinogen
    D. Factor II

The answer is D. Normal, aged serum contains coagulation factors VII, IX, X, XI, and XII, and normal aluminum hydroxide–adsorbed citrated plasma contains factors I, V, VIII, XI, and XII. In the APTT procedure, the reagents provide an activator (to ensure maximal activation), a phospholipid substitute for platelets (partial thromboplastin), and calcium chloride. Therefore, if an APTT were performed on a mixture of serum and adsorbed plasma, the factor that would need to be added for normal clot formation would be factor II, or prothrombin. (Brown, pp. 130–132, 146–150)

14. All of the following statements about hemoglobin S is (are) true except

    A. It is formed by substitution of valine for glutamic acid at the sixth position of the beta chain.
    B. It demonstrates altered electrophoretic mobility due to change of surface charge.
    C. It is freely soluble when fully oxygenated.
    D. It is formed by substitution of lysine for glutamic acid at the sixth position of the beta chain.

The answer is D. Hemoglobin S has valine substituted for glutamic acid at the sixth position on the beta chain. This amino acid substitution alters the surface charge, which changes the electrophoretic mobility. It is only when the oxygen tension is lowered that hemoglobin S crystals form and deform the red cells. (Henry)

15. The type of bone marrow specimen that is most valuable in estimating marrow cellularity and histologic structure is a

    A. Thin film of aspirated marrow
    B. Thick smear of aspirated marrow

C. Touch preparation of biopsied marrow

D. Sectioned preparation of biopsied marrow

The answer is D. The histologic architecture and cellularity of bone marrow are best evaluated in a sectioned biopsy preparation because the relation of cells to each other is preserved. Individual cells are best identified by thin films, thick smear, or touch preparations. (Williams et al.)

16. A physician requests that the laboratory establish a protocol for evaluation of iron-related anemias. All of the following test procedures should be included *except*

A. Bone marrow evaluation

B. Ferritin level

C. Red cell indices including the red cell distribution width

D. Serum iron and total iron-binding capacity (TIBC)

The answer is A. Iron deficiency anemias may have numerous causes and can be confused with other diseases such as thalassemia minor. It is important to determine cause and disease with as little trauma and cost to the patient as possible. The above tests can often give the necessary information without the need for a bone marrow aspiration. (Williams et al.)

17. The anomaly in which granulocytes have hyposegmented nuclei and markedly condensed nuclear chromatin is

A. Alder-Reilly

B. Chédiak-Higashi

C. Pelger-Huët

D. May-Hegglin

The answer is C. Granulocytes in the Pelger-Huët anomaly are characterized by hyposegmentation of their nuclei, which show marked condensation of nuclear chromatin. The abnormal nuclear maturation is presumed to be a reflection of abnormal nucleic acid metabolism, although the basic abnormality is unknown. Cytoplasmic maturation in these cells is normal. (Miale)

18. What erythrocyte morphology would probably be seen on a blood smear of a 50-year-old alcoholic with advanced cirrhosis?

A. Pseudomacrocytosis, acanthocytes, codocytes

B. Anisocytosis, microspherocytes, schistocytes

C. Macrocytosis, schistocytes, dacryocytes (teardrop cells)

D. Microcytosis, polychromasia, echinocytes

The answer is A. Pseudomacrocytosis is common in cirrhosis. The red cells appear larger than normal, but there is no increase in MCV or MCH. Both acanthocytes and codocytes may be seen in alcoholic cirrhosis as a result of abnormalities in plasma lipids that probably alter the lipid composition of the cell membrane. (Wintrobe)

19. While performing a differential on a peripheral blood smear, one encounters many schistocytes on the red cell morphology. One of the most common causes for these fragmented red cells is

A. Abnormal hemoglobin
B. Hemolytic anemia induced by *Clostridium* exotoxin
C. A leaky prosthetic heart valve
D. A high-titer cold agglutinin

The answer is C. Schistocytes are fragmented red cells that can be produced by the mechanical destruction caused by a leaky heart valve as the blood flows through. In assuming a variety of shapes, some of them may mimic other conditions. (Miale)

20. A nucleated erythrocyte containing diffuse blue or green granules when stained with Prussian blue stain is identified as a

A. Ringed sideroblast
B. Sideroblast
C. Pappenheimer cell
D. Siderocyte

The answer is B. Prussian blue stains iron-blue or green. Siderocytes, sideroblasts, and ringed sideroblasts are iron-containing erythrocytes. Sideroblasts are nucleated erythrocytes with diffuse iron. (Miale)

21. The half-life of labeled circulating granulocytes in normal peripheral blood has been estimated to be

A. 7 hr
B. 1 day
C. 3 days
D. 5 days

The answer is A. After the return of labeled neutrophils to their donor, the disappearance of labeled neutrophils from the blood shows a half-life of about 7 hr in most normal persons. (Wintrobe)

22. The following results are obtained on a bone marrow differential:

Early and mature neutrophils	30%
Eosinophils	1%
Basophils	0%
Lymphocytes	7%
Monocytes	1%
Plasmocytes	1%
Normoblasts	60%

What is the myeloid-erythroid (M:E) ratio?

A. 2:1
B. 1:2
C. 3:1
D. 1:5

The answer is B. The total percentage of myelocytic series (neutrophils, eosinophils, basophils) observed in relation to the total percentage of erythro-blastic series gives the M:E ratio. In the example given, the total percentage of myelocytic cells is 31%, and the total percentage of erythroblasts (normoblasts) is 60%; therefore, the M:E ratio is 1:2. (Williams et al.)

23. In severe idiopathic thrombocytopenic purpura (ITP), the viability of the platelets in the circulation is less than the normal viability of

A. 2 days
B. 10 days
C. 18 days
D. 22 days

The answer is B. Eight to 12 days are required for human platelets labeled with Cr^{51} to be cleared from the bloodstream. In each of several hundred patients with ITP, platelet life span was diminished. The shortest survival times were observed in the patients with the most severe thrombocytopenia. (Williams et al.)

24. On a hemoglobin electrophoresis pattern on cellulose acetate at pH 8.6, a band is present in the S region. What other laboratory test could be performed to help identify this hemoglobin?

A. Alkali denaturation
B. Hemoglobin solubility
C. Acid electrophoresis on agar, pH 6.0
D. Heat stability

The answer is C. Alkali denaturation is used for the differentiation of Hb F and Hb A, which are not in the Hb S region. Hemoglobin solubility is a screening procedure. Acid electrophoresis is a useful procedure for fractionation of various hemoglobins. At pH 6.0 to 6.2, it distinguishes Hb S from Hb D. Heat stability is a nonspecific test for unstable abnormal hemoglobins. (Wintrobe)

25. A patient with leukemia is undergoing a chemotherapeutic regimen that includes a drug that is antagonistic to folic acid metabolism. What type of erythrocytes may be produced as a result of using this drug?

A. Spherocytes
B. Microcytes
C. Codocytes
D. Macrocytes

The answer is D. Many of the chemotherapeutic agents have very toxic side effects. For example, the folic acid antagonists can result in megaloblastic maturation, and therefore production of macrocytes, especially if renal function is impaired. Because of this, it may be very important to determine the presence of macrocytes, which may appear before the MCV is elevated sufficiently to be considered abnormal. (Williams)

26. Blood is drawn from a patient who has a bacteremia caused by *Clostridium welchii*. The phlebotomist observes that the color of the blood appears to be mauve-lavender. Which abnormal hemoglobin would result in this type of discoloration of whole blood?

    A. Carboxyhemoglobin
    B. Sulfhemoglobin
    C. Methemoglobin
    D. Oxyhemoglobin

The answer is B. Patients with *C. welchii* have been reported to form sulfhemoglobin, which imparts a mauve-lavender cast to the blood sample. Carboxyhemoglobin contains carbon monoxide and is cherry-red. Methemoglobin is simply oxidized hemoglobin and is chocolate-brown in color. Oxyhemoglobin is normal hemoglobin with oxygen attached. (Henry)

27. Which of the following findings is *not* characteristic of aplastic anemia?

    A. Decreased reticulocyte count
    B. Increased Hb F
    C. Relative lymphocytosis
    D. Decreased erythropoietin

The answer is D. Aplastic anemia is characterized by decreased red cell count, white cell count, and platelet count. The leukopenia is usually due to decreased granulocytes; lymphocyte production is usually normal. The absolute reticulocyte count is below normal. Erythropoietin levels are higher in aplastic anemia than in other types of anemia with a similar hemoglobin level. The increased levels of fetal hemoglobin in patients with aplastic anemia has not been explained. (Williams et al.)

28. The Hb A_2 level is increased in beta thalassemia. This value may be artificially depressed in patients with beta thalassemia and

    A. Hereditary persistence of Hb F
    B. Hemolytic anemia
    C. Iron deficiency anemia
    D. Renal malfunction

The answer is C. Hb A_2 values may be artificially depressed in patients with beta thalassemia who have coexistent iron deficiency anemia. On institution of iron therapy, A_2 values increase the beta thalassemia range. (Williams et al.)

29. In milder forms of A-type G-6-PD deficiency, a drug-induced hemolytic episode may be self-limiting due to

    A. The increased red cell count
    B. A change in drug dosage
    C. The presence of many young red cells that have nearly normal G-6-PD levels
    D. The hemolytic episode having been drug-induced

The answer is C. In A-type G-6-PD deficiency, the hemolytic anemia is self-limiting. Young red cells produced in response to hemolysis have nearly normal G-6-PD levels and are resistant to hemolysis. Hemoglobin levels may return to normal even while some dosage of the drug is still being administered. (Williams et al.)

30. Megaloblastic anemias are characterized by all of the following *except*

    A. Dysynchronous cell maturation
    B. Hypochromasia
    C. Pancytopenia
    D. Macrocytic indices

The answer is B. Megaloblastic anemias are a group of anemias having a common pattern of morphologic and functional abnormalities. They are characterized by larger than normal cells with an unbalanced growth pattern. They are most often caused by vitamin B_{12} and folate deficiencies and result in pancytopenia. (Williams et al.)

31. When the interpretation of an erythrocyte survival curve indicates a half-life shorter than normal, one might also expect to observe all of the following *except*

    A. Decreased serum haptoglobin level
    B. Increased serum bilirubin
    C. Elevated reticulocyte count
    D. Decreased osmotic fragility

The answer is D. A shortened half-life indicates the presence of a hemolytic process. The accelerated rate of red cell sequestration produces increased bilirubin. Since haptoglobin is eliminated in the process, the serum level of this compound will be considerably reduced. Finally, the bone marrow response is to increase the rate of red cell production, thus increasing the reticulocyte count. (Wintrobe)

32. Chromium 51 can be used in the determination of

    A. Erythropoietin levels
    B. Erythrocyte survival times
    C. Vitamin B_{12} absorption studies
    D. G-6-PD levels

The answer is B. Radioactive chromium attaches to the beta chain of Hb A and the gamma chain of Hb F. It emits a high-energy gamma ray and allows radioactivity to be monitored easily. Therefore, it is the isotope of choice for determining red cell half-life. Radioactive cobalt is used in the Schilling test for vitamin B_{12} absorption, and radioactive iron is used in the determination of erythropoietin. The usual tests for G-6-PD levels do not use isotopes. (Wintrobe)

33. In the peripheral blood, chronic lymphocytic leukemia is characterized by

    A. A decreased number of mature lymphocytes
    B. Many large, reactive lymphocytes
    C. A predominance of lymphoblasts
    D. Many smudged cells

The answer is D. The peripheral blood smear in chronic lymphocytic leukemia shows a monotonous picture of small, mature lymphocytes. The neutrophil count is usually reduced. Particularly characteristic is the presence of many smudged cells, which is caused by the action of smearing and is due to the extreme mechanical fragility of the lymphocytes in this disease. (Miale)

34. Large platelets are commonly found in all of the following diseases *except*

    A. May-Hegglin anomaly
    B. Thrombocytopenia
    C. Myeloproliferative diseases
    D. Chronic liver disease

The answer is D. Large platelets are one of the characteristics of the May-Hegglin anomaly. In thrombocytopenia, the large platelets are presumed to be younger than usual, formed early as a compensatory mechanism, and in myeloproliferative disorders they are presumed to be due to maturation defect. They are not usually seen in chronic liver disease. (Miale)

35. Tests that can be used to quantitate Hb F include all of the following *except*

    A. Hemoglobin electrophoresis
    B. Kleihauer-Betke test
    C. Alkali denaturation
    D. Dithionite solubility

The answer is D. Hemoglobin electrophoresis separates and quantitates hemoglobins, including Hb F, on the basis of their migration in an electric field; the Kleihauer-Betke test detects and quantitates acid-resistant hemoglobin (F); and the alkali denaturation test quantitates alkali-resistant hemoglobin (F). The dithionite solubility test is used to detect and quantitate "insoluble" hemoglobins, such as Hb S and Hb C. (Henry)

36. A 6-year-old black boy with hepatosplenomegaly and a history of severe anemia has the following hematologic results:

WBC: 4.8×10^9/L
RBC: 2.5×10^{12}/L
Hb: 6.0 g/dl
Plt: 125.0×10^9/L
Retic: 205.0×10^9/L
Marked hypochromasia, anisocytosis, and poikilocytosis, with many target
  cells
20 nucleated RBCs per 100 WBCs

Additional studies reveal increased serum iron and increased Hb F. What is
the probable cause of these findings?

A. Aplastic anemia
B. Beta thalassemia major
C. Sickle cell anemia
D. Iron deficiency anemia

The answer is B. The hypochromic cells rule out aplastic anemia and sickle cell
anemia as a probable cause. The high serum iron rules out iron deficiency. The
morphology, history, and increase in Hb F and iron levels are all compatible
with a diagnosis of beta thalassemia. (Miale)

37. Relative polycythemia is caused by a decrease in the plasma portion of the
    blood. In relative polycythemia, all of the following are true *except*

    A. Hemoglobin and hematocrit are elevated.
    B. Peripheral blood smear usually shows normocytic, normochromic red
        cells.
    C. Number of cells per unit volume of blood is increased.
    D. Red cell mass is increased.

The answer is D. In relative polycythemia due to decreased plasma volume,
only the total plasma compartment of blood is affected. Therefore, although the
red count, hemoglobin, and hematocrit values reflect the decreased plasma
volume, the total red cell mass is unchanged, and the red cells are normocytic,
normochromic. (Brown)

38. Which of the following will cause the least inhibitory effect on the leuko-
    cyte alkaline phosphatase (LAP) stain?

    A. Collection of blood in EDTA
    B. Fingerstick blood smears collected 24 hr before staining
    C. Fingerstick blood smears fixed and stored at 0°C for 24 hr
    D. Fixed and stained fresh fingerstick smears cleaned with xylene

The answer is C. It is preferable to perform the LAP reaction immediately or to
fix films and store in the freezer. At room temperature, activity declines to 20%
below the original value at 24 hr. The stained granules fade if exposed to
organic solvents; therefore, avoid mounting media containing them and pro-

longed exposure to xylene or immersion oil. Enzyme activity diminishes rapidly in EDTA samples. (Henry)

39. Increased levels of Hb F have been associated with all the following *except*

    A. Paroxysmal nocturnal hemoglobinuria (PNH)
    B. Sideroblastic anemia
    C. Acute leukemia of childhood
    D. Iron deficiency anemia

The answer is D. When a differential diagnosis includes hemoglobinopathies and thalassemias, laboratory testing usually includes quantitation of Hb F and Hb A_2. Many diseases other than hemoglobinopathies are characterized by increased levels of Hb F. Increased Hb F has been found in some instances of pernicious anemia, aplastic anemia, PNH, refractory anemia, sideroblastic anemia, and childhood acute leukemias. (Miale, p. 633)

40. A patient's admission CBC shows the following data:

WBC:	8.9×10^9/L
RBC:	3.1×10^9/L
Hb:	9.1 g/dl
Hct:	27 L/L
Retic:	37%, uncorrected
RBC morphology:	polychromasia, moderate anisocytosis
Differential WBC count:	normal
Platelet estimate:	normal

CBCs performed at 48-hr intervals over a 2-week period show progressively lower Hb, Hct, and RBC levels with no significant changes in morphology. This appears to be a case of

    A. Decompensated hemolytic anemia
    B. Dyserythropoiesis
    C. Compensated hemolytic anemia
    D. Aplastic anemia

The answer is A. The fact that the anemia progressively worsens indicates that it is decompensated; if the marrow were successfully compensating for the loss, the Hb, Hct, and RBC levels would have leveled off. The presence of abundant reticulocytes rules out dyserythropoiesis. (Miale)

41. The presence of many stained cells compared to unstained ghost cells on a Kleihauer-Betke stain is compatible with all of the following *except*

    A. Thalassemia
    B. Cord blood

C. Hereditary persistence of fetal hemoglobin
D. Sickle cell trait

The answer is D. The Kleihauer-Betke test differentiates between acid-resistant Hb F and other hemoglobins, such as A, that are eluted in an acid buffer. The presence of many cells containing Hb F could be due to thalassemia, hereditary persistence of fetal hemoglobin, or cord blood. (Henry)

42. Confirmatory testing for infectious mononucleosis includes all of the following *except*

A. Heterophile antibody test
B. Examination of blood smear for reactive lymphocytes
C. Epstein-Barr (E-B) antibody titer
D. Antistreptolysin O (ASO) titer

The answer is D. Patients with infectious mononucleosis usually have a positive E-B antibody titer, a heterophile titer, and reactive lymphocytes on their peripheral smear. An ASO titer is often elevated in patients who have had group A streptococcal infections. (Williams et al.)

43. A peripheral blood smear contains 80% blast cells, which stain positively with Sudan black B and peroxidase. This result is indicative of

A. Acute lymphocytic leukemia
B. Acute undifferentiated leukemia
C. Chronic granulocytic leukemia
D. Acute granulocytic leukemia

The answer is D. Lymphoid cells characteristically do not stain with Sudan black B and peroxidase. Undifferentiated cells have not matured enough to stain positively with either Sudan black B or peroxidase. Chronic granulocytic leukemia does not show 80% blast cells (unless the patient is in a blastic crisis); therefore, this picture is most indicative of acute granulocytic leukemia, in which the blasts often stain positively with Sudan black B and peroxidase. (Williams, et al.)

44. A CBC on a blood sample is processed on a Coulter S Plus system; the instrument has been correctly calibrated and is in control. Repeated values (× 3) on this sample reveal:

RBC: $3.72 \times 10^6/\mu l$
Hct: 0.32 L/L
Hb: 12.0 g/dl
MCV: 86 fl
MCH: 32 pg
MCHC: 37.5 g/dl

The most likely explanation for these results is

A. A macrocytic anemia
B. Hereditary spherocytosis
C. A high titer of cold agglutinins
D. A high reticulocyte count

The answer is B. In hereditary spherocytosis, the MCHC is often increased (greater than 36%) because of a decrease in cell surface area. Other indices are not significantly affected. (Henry)

45. The aberrant cell in multiple myeloma is a

A. Megaloblast
B. Myeloblast
C. Plasma cell
D. Reactive lymphocyte

The answer is C. The most characteristic finding in the bone marrow of patients with myeloma is an increase in morphologically abnormal plasma cells. (Williams et al.)

46. Which antibody is basic to the formation of an LE cell?

A. Antideoxyribonucleic acid (anti-DNA)
B. Antideoxyribonucleoprotein (anti-DNP)
C. Antinuclear histones (extractable)
D. Antiribonucleic acid (anti-RNA)

The answer is B. Anti-DNP is found most commonly in systemic lupus erythematosus, but also in other collagen diseases, including rheumatoid arthritis. (Henry; Williams et al.)

47. Which French, American, and British (FAB) classification is represented by the following data?

Both granulocytic and monocytic differentiation are present in the peripheral blood and bone marrow.
Blasts are Sudan black-positive.
Blasts are alpha-naphthyl-acetate–positive.

A. M1
B. M3
C. M4
D. M5

The answer is C. The French, American and British classification of leukemia separates the acute leukemias into myeloid and nonmyeloid categories. Additional subdivision into six myeloid and three lymphoid types is done according to cell line differentiation, cell maturation, and morphology. The M4 category represents myelomonocytic leukemia. Both granulocytic and monocytic differentiation are present in the peripheral blood and bone marrow. Cytochemically, the blast cells from this leukemia are both Sudan black B–positive and alpha-naphthyl-acetate–positive. (Henry)

48. The differentiation of the acute leukemias is of major concern due to the various prognostic and therapeutic variables. When the bone marrow smear is primarily blastic in nature, appropriate laboratory procedures include all of the following *except*

   A. Cytogenetic studies
   B. Examination of blastic morphology
   C. Cytochemical evaluation
   D. Determination of the myeloid-erythroid (M:E) ratio

The answer is D. Cytochemical reactions should be used as an adjunct to standard morphology. The association of chromosomal abnormalities with leukemia has been well established. (Miale)

49. As the supervisory technologist, you are asked to review a Wright's-stained blood smear, which shows nuclear pyknosis in many of the leukocytes and a moderate number of crenated red cells. Which of the following is the most probable cause for these morphologic changes?

   A. Smear made from 1-hr-old oxalated blood
   B. Smear made from 1-hr-old EDTA blood
   C. Excessive pressure applied when making smear from blood in tip of vacuum tube needle
   D. Smear made using fresh capillary blood

The answer is A. The effect of oxalates on cell morphology, especially on leukocytes, is almost immediate, whereas cells in EDTA blood are stable for up to 2 hr. Nonanticoagulated blood should show no cellular artifacts with proper preparation of smear. (Brown)

50. A CBC is performed using the following instruments:

   Coleman Jr. spectrophotometer: hemoglobin
   IL microcentrifuge: hematocrit
   Coulter Z_F: cell counts (RBC and WBC)
   Calculated indices
     MCV: 93 fl
     MCH: 28 pg
     MCHC: 30.1 g/dl

The blood film reveals a few normocytic, normochromic red cells with a large population of markedly microcytic, hypochromic cells. These data indicate that the

  A. RBC count is invalidly low.
  B. Hemoglobin is invalidly high.
  C. Hematocrit is invalidly high.
  D. RBC count is invalidly high.

The answer is A. For the population of red cells described, both the MCV and MCH appear to be invalidly high. Common to both of these calculations is the RBC count. If the RBC count is falsely low, both the MCV and MCH will be invalidly elevated. (Henry)

References

Brown, B. A. *Hematology: Principles and Procedures* (5th ed.). Philadelphia: Lea & Febiger, 1988.

Diggs, L. W., et al. *The Morphology of Human Blood Cells* (5th ed.). Chicago: Abbott Laboratories, 1985.

Harker, L. *Hemostasis Manual* (3rd ed.). Philadelphia: Davis, 1983.

Henry, J. B. (Ed.). *Clinical Diagnosis and Management by Laboratory Methods* (17th ed.). Philadelphia: Saunders, 1984.

Lee, L. W. *Elementary Principles of Laboratory Instruments* (5th ed.). St. Louis: Mosby, 1983.

Miale, J. B. *Laboratory Medicine: Hematology* (6th ed.). St. Louis: Mosby, 1982.

Platt, W. R. *Color Atlas and Textbook of Hematology* (2nd ed.). Philadelphia: Lippincott, 1979.

Sirridge, M., and Shannon, R. *Laboratory Evaluation of Hemostasis and Thrombosis* (3rd ed.). Philadelphia: Lea & Febiger, 1983.

Williams, W. J., et al. *Hematology* (3rd ed.). New York: McGraw-Hill, 1983.

Wintrobe, M. M. *Clinical Hematology* (8th ed.). Philadelphia: Lea & Febiger, 1981.

Section Editor
Susan Beck, M.S.

Contributors
Judy Adams, Ph.D.
Ralph M. Aloisi, Ph.D.
Deborah Anderson
L.B. Bachert
Michael A. Beard, Ed.D.
Margaret B. Boone
Diane Breen
Suzanne H. Butch, M.A.
Sandra Carter, M.S.
Joan E. Charbonneau, M.S.
Beverly Fiorella, M.A.
Dorothy M. Floyd, M.A.
David Fowler
Vahe Ghazarian
Jo Martha Glushko
Mary M. Gourley
Helen Hallgren, M.S.
Nancy Jensen, M.S.
Karen R. Karni, Ph.D.
Laurie Langen
Susan J. Leclair, M.S.
Carol L. Libby
Daryl Marcoux
Kenneth T. Maehara, Ph.D.
Kathryn Massey
Carol McCoy, M.S.
Roberta Montgomery
Clareyse Nelson
Melanie Palmer
Kathryn Petershagen
S. M. H. Qadri
Marion Reid
Joseph Rizzo, M.S.
Susan Salentine
Alice Smith-Floss, M.A.
Kim Stecher-Northcut
E. Camellia St. John, M.Ed.
Joyce Trembath, M.S.
Theresa Vincent
Mary Margaret Webb
Sherry Wilkening
Naoum Yioras
Kay Zelenski, Ph.D.

CLT Review Questions

1. In humans, what organ is considered responsible for producing T lymphocytes?

   A. Bursa of Fabricius
   B. Liver
   C. Spleen
   D. Thymus

The answer is D. The thymus, located behind the sternum in humans, is an
organ once thought to be vestigial (of no importance, somewhat like the appen-
dix), largely because it begins to atrophy when humans near the age of 10. It is
now known that the thymus, which is essential for immunity, is responsible for
the production of lymphocytes involved in cell-mediated immune responses (T
lymphocytes). (Bellanti)

2. Cells that synthesize antibody are

   A. Macrophages
   B. Immature T lymphocytes
   C. Mature B lymphocytes
   D. Mature T lymphocytes

The answer is C. Humoral immunity is due to circulating immunoglobulins.
The cells that synthesize immunoglobulins are mature B lymphocytes; plasma
cells are the most mature forms. (Henry)

3. Which of the following functions is characteristic of the *cellular* immune
   system?

   A. Rejection of transplants
   B. Activation of complement
   C. Immediate hemolytic transfusion reactions
   D. Immunoglobulin production

The answer is A. The immune system is composed of the cellular and humoral
immune systems. The cellular immune system, which consists of T lymphocytes, is responsible for cellular immunity, tissue graft rejection, delayed hypersensitivity reactions, and immunologic surveillance. (Bellanti)

4. In the diagram below of a typical immune response, curve 2 represents

   A. IgG immunoglobulins
   B. A primary response
   C. Antibodies that agglutinate red cells directly
   D. IgM immunoglobulins

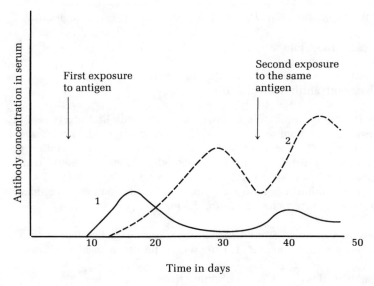

Time in days

The answer is A. Once a person has reached immunologic maturity, the response to an antigenic stimulus can be fairly well predicted. Curve 1 represents a primary response, which tends to elicit IgM (direct agglutination) antibodies. Curve 2 is the secondary, or anamnestic (remembering), response, which tends to cause a proliferation of IgG (coating) antibodies. (Bryant)

5. Which phrase best describes the term *alloantigen?*

    A. A synonym for hapten
    B. An antigen that reacts with antibodies from individuals within the same species
    C. An antigen from an individual that reacts against that individual's own antibodies.
    D. An antigen from an individual of one species that reacts with antibodies produced by individuals of another species

The answer is B. The following are basic definitions in immunology:

Hapten: a low-molecular-weight substance (<5000) that rarely stimulates the production of antibodies, but which can react with antibody if present. A hapten can induce an immune response if coupled to a carrier protein.

Alloantigen: an antigen that reacts with antibodies from within the same species. Correspondingly, an alloantibody is an antibody produced in response to antigens contained within the tissues of another of the same species (e.g., human transfusion may produce alloantibodies).

Autoantibody: an antibody produced in response to an antigen possessed by the same individual.

Heterophile antibody (xenoantibody): an antibody produced in one species that reacts with antigen from another species (e.g., the antibodies found in infectious mononucleosis). (Stites et al.)

6. Which of the following characteristics is typical of IgG immunoglobulins?

    A. React best at room temperature
    B. Are naturally occurring
    C. Are sensitive to treatment with dithiothreitol (DTT)
    D. React best with antihuman globulin

The answer is D. The IgG molecule is an immune antibody that reacts best at 37°C. It is resistant to treatment with sulfhydryl compounds such as 2-mercaptoethanol and DTT, whereas IgM antibodies are reduced by these reagents. Antibodies of the IgG class often react with antigenic determinants present on red blood cells but do not demonstrate a visible reaction. Consequently, antihuman globulin is required to produce agglutination. (*Technical Manual of the American Association of Blood Banks*)

7. Below are listed classes of immunoglobulins and characteristics of these classes. Select the immunoglobulin for which no characteristic is listed.

Immunoglobulin class	Characteristic
IgA	Passes the placenta from mother to fetus
IgG	Is a pentamer
IgE	Binds to mast cells
IgM	Fixes complement

    A. IgA
    B. IgG
    C. IgE
    D. IgM

The answer is A. None of the characteristics listed are associated with the IgA class of antibody. Only the IgG class crosses the placental barrier, and only IgG and IgM fix complement. IgM is the largest of all the classes, with a molecular weight of 900,000 daltons, and is arranged in the form of a pentamer. The IgE molecule is a reaginic antibody that binds to mast cells by the Fc portion and is associated with immediate hypersensitivity reactions (type I). IgA aggregation activates the complement cascade by way of the alternate pathway. (*Technical Manual of the American Association of Blood Banks*)

8. Antibodies in which of the following immunoglobulin classes are capable of binding complement?

    A. IgA
    B. IgD
    C. IgE
    D. IgG

The answer is D. The five immunoglobulin classes—IgG, IgM, IgA, IgD, IgE—are distinguished primarily by their amino acids in the constant region of their heavy classes. They also differ in other characteristics: molecular weight, electrophoretic mobility, concentration in serum, ability to cross the placenta, and ability to fix complement. To date, only IgG and IgM have been characterized as able to fix complement. Therefore, IgA, IgD, and IgE are not considered capable of binding complement. (Bryant)

9. The results of an agglutination test using successive dilutions of patient serum are shown below. What do the result in tubes 1 to 5 represent?

Tube No.

1	2	3	4	5	6	7	8	9	10
1:2	1:4	1:8	1:16	1:32	1:64	1:128	1:256	1:512	Antigen control
0	0	0	0	0	+	+	+	+	0

Key: + = agglutination; 0 = no agglutination.

A. Prozone due to antigen excess
B. Prozone due to antibody excess
C. Activation of complement sequence
D. Error in techniques; these results cannot occur when the agglutination procedure is performed correctly

The answer is B. These results represent the classic prozone phenomenon due to antibody excess. It is thought that excess of antibody, in relation to antigen, prevents the formation of a lattice. (Stites et al., p. 241)

10. Two procedures, the RPR and FTA-ABS, are used for screening and confirmation of syphilis because

A. The RPR test is specific; the FTA-ABS test is sensitive.
B. The RPR test is sensitive; the FTA-ABS test is specific.
C. Both tests are highly sensitive.
D. Both tests are highly specific.

The answer is B. The screening tests for syphilis (of which the RPR is an example) are nontreponemal antigen tests. They are relatively sensitive, but may lack specificity. Confirmatory tests (of which the FTA-ABS is an example) use a treponemal antigen and are more specific than the screening tests for treponemal antibody. (Henry, pp. 1140–1142)

11. Which of the tests listed below is not a third-generation test for the detection of HB$_s$Ag?

A. Latex agglutination
B. Radioimmunoassay
C. Reversed passive hemagglutination
D. Enzyme-linked immunosorbent assay

The answer is A. The Bureau of Biologics requires that testing for hepatitis B surface antigen (HB$_s$Ag) be performed using reagents and techniques licensed by the Food and Drug Administration as "third-generation" tests. These tests include radioimmunoassay, enzyme-linked immunosorbent assay, and reversed passive hemagglutination. (*Technical Manual of the American Association of Blood Banks*)

12. Davidsohn's differential test for infectious mononucleosis has been modified into a rapid plate test. Horse cells, which are more sensitive than sheep cells, are used as the indicator system. The test is set up as follows:

    Left side of slide: patient serum + guinea pig kidney reagent + horse cells
    Right side of slide: patient serum + beef erythrocytes + horse cells

    The reactions look as follows:

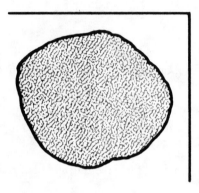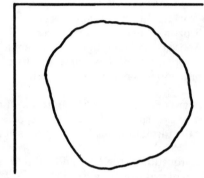

    These findings indicate

    A. Normal serum
    B. Infectious hepatitis
    C. Serum sickness
    D. Infectious mononucleosis

The answer is D. On the left side of the slide, the patient serum is not absorbed by guinea pig kidney. Therefore, the person's heterophile antibodies are not neutralized and can react with horse cells to give agglutination. This is a positive reaction for infectious mononucleosis. On the right side of the slide, the patient serum is absorbed by beef erythrocytes. Therefore, no antibody is left to react with horse cells, and no agglutination results. (Henry)

13. Which of the following statements is true regarding C-reactive protein (CRP)?

    A. It is commonly found in healthy persons.
    B. It remains in the serum after an inflammatory process has subsided.
    C. It can be elevated in postoperative patients.
    D. It is diagnostic for active rheumatic fever.

The answer is C. CRP, not an antibody, is a substance produced by the liver in a variety of inflammatory, necrotic, and infectious diseases. It reacts with anti-CRP in a precipitation reaction. CRP is present in the sera of patients with acute myocardial infarcts, active rheumatic fever, and other infectious diseases. The presence of CRP is not diagnostic for a specific disease but indicates necrosis and inflammation of numerous origins. Thus CRP can be seen postoperatively, or even in pregnant women. CRP is not found in healthy persons, and it disappears rapidly following recovery from disease. (Henry)

14. Which of the following is true of the classic antistreptolysin O (ASO) test?

    A. This procedure is a neutralization test.
    B. Streptolysin O combines with antibody, and the complex activates complement, which is added to the test system, giving hemolysis.
    C. Controls used should show the streptolysin control with no lysis and the red cell control with complete lysis.
    D. Hemolysis of red cells indicates the presence of antibody.

The answer is A. The ASO test is a neutralization test: antistreptolysin O, present in a person with a group A streptococcal infection, neutralizes the reagent streptolysin, making it unavailable to lyse reagent red cells. Complement is not involved. Therefore, if a person's serum contains ASO antibodies, these will combine with the antigen (streptolysin) and neutralize its hemolytic activity. The streptolysin control should show complete lysis, and the red cell control should show no lysis. (Bryant)

15. Which of the following statements is true regarding anti-I?

    A. It is associated with hemolytic disease of the newborn.
    B. It is usually a cold agglutinin.
    C. It reacts best at 37°C.
    D. It is not found in the serum of I-positive individuals.

The answer is B. Anti-I is generally an IgM immunoglobulin, reacting best at 4°C. It is associated with atypical pneumonia (caused by *Mycoplasma pneumoniae*) as well as cold autoimmune hemolytic anemia. It is reactive with most I-positive adult cells when the tests are run at cold temperatures. Although most adults are I-positive, a few are not; these i_{adult} persons can be expected to have anti-I as an alloantibody. (*Technical Manual of the American Association of Blood Banks*)

16. A common test kit for rheumatoid factor (RF) contains a saline diluent, positive and negative controls, and an IgG-latex particle complex. In this procedure, which of the following statement(s) is (are) true?

    A. The RF in patient serum primarily represents IgG immunoglobulin.
    B. The test is specific for rheumatoid arthritis.
    C. RF inhibits the agglutination of the latex particles.
    D. A positive reaction is indicated by agglutination of the latex particles.

The answer is D. Most tests for RF are passive hemagglutination procedures, in which antigen (IgG) is linked to latex particles (or sheep RBCs). RF, an IgM, appears to be a by-product of rheumatoid arthritis and will react with this IgG-particle complex. Specifically, RF in the patient's serum combines (by its Fab region) to the Fc region of the IgG molecule added. Since the IgG is passively attached to latex, the latex particles are agglutinated.

The test is not specific; false positives are seen in syphilis, lupus erythematosus, and other diseases. Nor is there correlation between titer and disease severity. (Henry)

17. Which of the following is most likely to cause a *false* negative pregnancy test by immunoassay?

    A. Specific gravity (< 1.010)
    B. Proteinuria (> 1 g/24 hr)
    C. Positive glucose
    D. pH (< 7.5)

The answer is A. False positive results in immunoassays such as hemagglutination inhibition or direct latex particle agglutination may result from a variety of factors, such as increased luteinizing hormone in menopausal women; drugs such as promethazine or methadone; and proteinuria. In contrast, false negative results can result from "dilute" urine (i.e., with very low specific gravity indicating lack of concentration of human chorionic gonadotropin) as well as from early pregnancy, ectopic pregnancy, or threatened abortion. (Henry)

18. Testing for HLA antigens is useful in

    A. Classifying acute leukemias
    B. Selecting donors for cryoprecipitate
    C. Paternity testing
    D. Testing for non-A, non-B hepatitis

The answer is C. Testing for HLA antigens is useful for assessing histocompatibility for organ transplantation, in paternity testing, and for selecting platelet or granulocyte donors. HLA typing is also done to determine the association between HLA type and certain diseases. It is not done for donations of cryoprecipitate, for classification of acute leukemias, or as a test to detect hepatitis. (*Technical Manual of the American Association of Blood Banks*)

19. Which of the serologic methods listed below is commonly used to detect rubella antibodies?

    A. Immunoelectrophoresis
    B. Latex agglutination
    C. Hemagglutination inhibition
    D. Precipitation

The answer is C. Screening for immune status is normally performed by determining levels of passive hemagglutination and hemagglutination inhibition antibodies. Both procedures measure antibodies that remain in the bloodstream for years. (Henry)

20. Below are the results of the physical examination of a female blood donor:

Last donation	3 months ago	Blood pressure	170/90 mm Hg
Age	65 years	Weight	112 lb
Hb	12.8 g/dl	Temperature	38°C
Pulse	95/min		

How many of the given values fall outside the acceptable limits set by the American Association of Blood Banks (AABB)?

A. None
B. One
C. Two
D. Three

The answer is B. Although several values are close to the limits, only one value falls outside the acceptable limit: the temperature must not exceed 37.5C. Other limits are:

Last donation: 8 weeks ago (minimum time interval)
Age: between 17 and 65 years (less than 66)
Hb: 12.5 g/dl—women; 13.5 g/dl—men
Pulse: between 50 and 100 with no pathologic cardiac irregularities
Blood pressure: systolic between 90 and 180 mm Hg
Weight: greater than 110 lb for a full unit to be drawn

(*Technical Manual of the American Association of Blood Banks*)

21. The blood group that reacts *least* strongly with anti-H lectin is

A. A_2
B. B
C. O
D. A_1B

The answer is D. Anti-H lectin reacts with cells in the following order of decreasing reactivity:

$O>A_2>A_2B>B>A_1>A_1B$

(*Technical Manual of the American Association of Blood Banks*)

22. Antibodies in the Rh system typically

    A. React better at 37°C than at room temperature
    B. Tend to be saline agglutinins
    C. Do not react with enzyme-treated cells
    D. Bind complement and cause in vitro hemolysis

The answer is A. Most antibodies in the Rh system result from immunization from either pregnancy or transfusion. They tend to be IgG, reacting best at 37°C in high protein or with antiglobulin or enzyme procedures. They rarely bind complement. (*Technical Manual of the American Association of Blood Banks*)

23. A patient has the phenotype O, CDEe. If transfused with blood from six donors who are group O, Rh-positive, this patient "theoretically" could produce the antibody(ies)

    A. Anti-D
    B. Anti-C
    C. None; the patient is Rh-positive
    D. Anti-c

The answer is D. Persons can build alloantibodies to antigens they do not possess. This patient, who has antigens C, D, E, and e, could produce anti-c if transfused with blood containing the c antigens. The chances of being transfused with blood with this c antigen is high since 31% of the white population and 9% of the black population are CDe/cde. (*Technical Manual of the American Association of Blood Banks*)

24. A patient is typed as group O, Rh-positive and crossmatched with 5 units of blood. The patient's antibody screening test and one compatibility test show agglutination in the antiglobulin phase. All other test results are negative on initial spin and at 37°C. The most probable antibody is

    A. Anti-I
    B. Anti-K
    C. Anti-M
    D. Anti-k

The answer is B. Anti-I and anti-M, which react at room temperature and below, are eliminated. Although anti-k is expected to react in the antiglobulin phase, it is directed against a high-incidence antigen. In its presence, all donor units would be expected to be incompatible. The optimal phase for anti-K reactivity is the antiglobulin phase. Although anti-K would be expected to give an incompatible crossmatch in one of 10 cases, in this instance its occurrence in one of five crossmatches is still probable. (*Technical Manual of the American Association of Blood Banks*)

25. Choose the list of four antibodies in which all generally react strongly at 4°C.

A. Anti-A, anti-P_1, anti-Le^a, anti-M
B. Anti-B, anti-K, anti-I, anti-Fy^a
C. Anti-H, anti-S, anti-Jk^a, anti-Le^b
D. Anti-PP$_1$P^k, anti-Lu^b, anti-Yt^a, anti-f

The answer is A. Antibodies that usually react strongly at 4°C are anti-A, anti-B, anti-H, anti-P_1, anti-PP$_1$P^k, anti-Le^b, anti-I, and anti-M. A few specimens of anti-S have been found to react well at 4°C. Antibodies that in general do not react at 4°C are anti-K, anti-Lu^b, anti-Jk^a, anti-Yt^a, anti-Fy^a, and anti-f (anti-Rh6). (*Technical Manual of the American Association of Blood Banks*)

26. Which is true of anti-M and anti-N?

    A. Are able to agglutinate cells in a saline medium
    B. React optimally at 37°C
    C. Are likely to cause hemolytic disease of the newborn
    D. React with enzyme-treated cells

The answer is A. Anti-M and anti-N are most often naturally occurring antibodies. They react best at room temperature or below and can agglutinate cells in a saline medium. They are more likely to react well with homozygous than with heterozygous cells and are seldom implicated in hemolytic transfusion reactions or hemolytic disease of the newborn. (*Technical Manual of the American Association of Blood Banks*)

27. All of the following are the statements concerning the Lewis blood group system *except*

    A. The antigens are primarily in the plasma and adsorb onto red cells.
    B. Lewis antibodies can be implicated in hemolytic disease of the newborn.
    C. Lewis antibodies can be neutralized in vivo.
    D. Cord blood is generally Le^a- and Le^b-negative.

The answer is B. Since IgM Lewis antibodies do not cross the placenta and Lewis antigens are poorly developed at birth, the antibodies in the Lewis system are not involved in hemolytic disease of the newborn. (*Technical Manual of the American Association of Blood Banks*)

28. The single most important serologic procedure in immunohematology is probably the

    A. Antiglobulin test (AGT)
    B. Titer for antibody strength
    C. Absorption-elution test
    D. Enzyme technique

The answer is A. The AGT has a wide range of applications including antibody detection and identification and crossmatch techniques. The AGT detects many IgG antibodies that do not react in saline or high protein media or react weakly in these media. It also detects antibodies that bind complement but may not be capable of binding to red cells in sufficient amounts to give a positive result. The AGT is also used to detect the in vivo coating of red blood cells with antibody or complement (direct antiglobulin test). (Pittiglio)

29. Group O, Rh_o-positive cells are used for antibody screening tests because

    A. Anti-A and Anti-B do not react with O cells.
    B. Anti-A_1 is detected using O cells.
    C. Most recipients are O, Rh-positive
    D. Weak A or B subtypes react with O cells.

The answer is A. O cells are selected to avoid interference from antibodies from the ABO system and to contain as many common red cell antigens as possible. Rh-positive cells are used to increase the likelihood of detecting unexpected anti-D. Anti-A_1 is not detected with O cells but is detected with A_1 cells. Weak A or B subtypes do not react with O cells (both represent antigen systems, rather than antigen plus antibody). (*Technical Manual of the American Association of Blood Banks*)

30. Both direct and indirect antiglobulin techniques require thorough washing. The following considerations are important for all procedures that use antiglobulin serum, *except*

    A. Washing is performed in as short a period of time as possible.
    B. Antiglobulin serum can be added any time up to 40 min after completion of washing.
    C. The volume of wash saline should fill the tube at least three-quarters full.
    D. The cell button should be fully resuspended in the residual saline after decanting and before addition of wash saline.

The answer is B. It is important that the antiglobulin serum be added immediately following completion of washing. If this is not done, cell-bound IgG may detach from the red cells and remain free in the fluid medium. These unbound molecules can inhibit the antiglobulin serum when it is added and, therefore, give a false negative reaction. (*Technical Manual of the American Association of Blood Banks*)

31. IgM antibodies directed against red cell antigens characteristically are

    A. Reactive at 37°C
    B. Not usually associated with hemolytic transfusion reaction or hemolytic disease of the newborn
    C. Clinically important is most instances
    D. Best demonstrated with antihuman globulin (AHG)

The answer is B. IgM antibodies react best at room temperature or below and are seldom associated with hemolytic transfusion reactions (perhaps because of their optimal reaction temperature). IgM antibodies may also occur transiently in the serum of patients or donors without stimulation by transfusion or pregnancy. AHG is not usually required to demonstrate their activity. (*Technical Manual of the American Association of Blood Banks*)

32. Proteolytic enzymes may enhance certain hemagglutination reactions. Which of the following groups of antigens show enhanced agglutination with the use of enzymes?

    A. M, N, D, e
    B. Jk^a, Jk^b, C, E
    C. Fy^a, Fy^b, Lu^a, Lu^b
    D. Fy^a, Jk^b, Lu^a, S

The answer is B. Enzyme techniques strengthen the reactions of certain antibodies, most notably those in the Rh and Kidd systems. Option B contains antigens from these two systems. The other options contain antigens that have been destroyed by enzymes, such as those in the Duffy and MNSs systems. (Henry)

33. From the abbreviated cell panel depicted below, determine the most probable antibody or antibodies in the patient's serum.

Panel cell No.	Known antigens									Test Results		
	C	D	E	c	e	K	k	M	N	IS	37°C	AHG
1	+	+	+	+	0	0	+	0	+	1+	2+	3+
2	0	+	0	+	+	0	+	+	0	0	0	0
3	0	+	+	+	0	0	+	+	0	1+	2+	4+
4	+	+	0	0	+	+	+	+	+	0	0	0
5	0	0	0	+	+	0	+	+	0	0	0	0
Autocontrol										0	0	0

Key: IS = initial spin; AHG = antihuman globulin.

    A. Anti-k
    B. Anti-e
    C. Anti-E
    D. Anti-e and C

The answer is C. From the panel antigens shown, possible antibodies are anti-C, D, E, c, e, K, k, M, and N. One first looks for negative results to rule out corresponding antibodies that would have given positive results. For example, there are no reactions of patient serum with cell 2. Since these cells contain D, c, e, k, and M antigens, corresponding antibodies must be absent or a positive reaction would have occurred. This gives the following pattern of antibody elimination: anti-C, D̸, E, c̸, e̸, K, k̸, M̸, and N. Only anti-C, E, K, and N remain. Since cell 4 also gives no results, the following are also eliminated: anti-C̸, E, K̸, and N̸, leaving anti-E. This also is the pattern seen with anti-E. Cell 5 is also negative, but this does not rule out additional antibodies.

E antigen is found only on cells 1 and 3, which are the only cells that give results with this serum. Anti-E also gives enhanced results at 37°C incubation and with AHG (*Technical Manual of the American Association of Blood Banks*)

34. What is the fundamental purpose of the crossmatch?

   A. Detect recipient antibodies that are directed against donor red cell antigens
   B. Prove that a recipient does, or does not, have an unexpected antibody in the serum
   C. Verify that the donor and recipient are Rh-identical
   D. Prevent immunization of the recipient

The answer is A. The crossmatch provides considerable safety in transfusion services. It can test to see that the ABO groups of recipient and donor are compatible, as in giving A blood to an A recipient or O blood to an A recipient. It can also determine whether the patient has detectable, unexpected antibodies directed against donor cells.

However, the crossmatch *cannot* prove that a recipient has no unexpected antibodies, nor can it guarantee that immunizations will not occur. In the latter instance, for example, an Rh-positive donor can give a compatible crossmatch with an Rh-negative recipient; however, the Rh-positive cells, when transfused, may immunize the recipient to produce anti-D. The crossmatch does not verify that the donor and recipient are Rh-identical. (*Technical Manual of the American Association of Blood Banks*)

35. Which of the following incompatibilities will the crossmatch (saline, albumin, antiglobulin test) usually detect? In each situation, no other unexpected antibodies are noted.

   A. O patient, mistyped as A; donor is A
   B. Rh-negative patient, mistyped as Rh-positive but having no unexpected antibodies; donor is Rh-positive.
   C. Patient with AHG reacting anti-Jk^a; donor is Jk(a−b+)
   D. Rh-positive patient with no unexpected antibodies; donor is Rh-negative

The answer is A. In option A the O patient has anti-A, which will react with the A cells of the donor. Although the patient in option B is Rh-negative, he or she has no anti-D to react with the D antigen of donor cells. In option C, the patient has an anti-Jk^a but the donor unit is negative for the Jk^a antigen. In option D the Rh-positive patient with no unexpected antibodies would be expected to give a compatible crossmatch with Rh-negative cells. (*Technical Manual of the American Association of Blood Banks*)

36. If the antiglobulin phase of the crossmatch is omitted, which of the following antibodies would probably *not* be detected?

A. Anti-K
B. Anti-A
C. Anti-P$_1$
D. Anti-N

The answer is A. Both antibodies of the Kell system, anti-K and anti-k, react best using antiglobulin. The same is true of anti-Jk^a and anti-Fy^a. Therefore these antibodies could be missed (not detected) if the antiglobulin phase were omitted. Anti-A, anti-P$_1$, and anti-N react best at cold temperatures and would be detected on immediate spin. (*Technical Manual of the American Association of Blood Banks*)

37. Which of the following would be an acceptable alternative for a blood transfusion if ABO type-specific blood was not available?

A. Group A recipient with group B donor
B. Group B recipient with group AB donor
C. Group O recipient with group A donor
D. Group AB recipient with group B donor

The answer is D. The major crossmatch uses patient serum with donor cells. In option A the A recipient has anti-B, which would react with the B cells of the donor. In option B the B recipient has anti-A, which would react with the A antigenic sites of the AB donor. In option C the group O recipient has anti-A and anti-B; the anti-A would react with the A cells of the donor. In option D, the AB recipient has neither anti-A nor anti-B; therefore, there are no antibodies in the ABO system to react with the B cells of the donor. Group A, B, or O blood can be given to an AB recipient, but only one of these types should be used for a given recipient if possible. (*Technical Manual of the American Association of Blood Banks*)

38. Choose the preferred criteria for donor units when issuing uncrossmatched blood for a patient who is bleeding profusely.

A. ABO- and Rh-specific
B. ABO-specific, Rh-negative
C. ABO- and Rh-compatible
D. Group O, Rh-negative

The answer is A. In emergency situations, blood may be issued that is neither typed nor crossmatched. If there is time for typing, blood that is type-specific (e.g., A-positive to A-positive) should be given. If blood that is type-specific is not available in sufficient quantity, type-compatible blood (e.g., O-negative to A-positive) may be given. Although ABO-specific blood that is Rh-negative (e.g., A-negative to A person, Rh status not determined) may be given, or, in dire emergencies, group O, Rh-negative blood may be given to one whose ABO and Rh status is not determined, it is still preferable to give ABO- and Rh-specific blood whenever possible. (*Technical Manual of the American Association of Blood Banks*)

39. A physician calls to notify a hospital that an accident victim, in shock, will probably need at least 5 units of packed red blood cells STAT on arrival. Considering the inventory of most blood bank laboratories, it would be easiest to find blood of the patient's own type, if this patient were

    A. A-negative
    B. B-positive
    C. O-positive
    D. AB-negative

The answer is C. The great majority of the population in the United States is Rh_o-positive. Group O is the most common ABO group in the United States, and group A is a close second. Of the choices listed, it would be easiest to find adequate amounts of O-positive blood for transfusion of this patient. (*Technical Manual of the American Association of Blood Banks*)

40. A patient who has repeated severe nonhemolytic febrile transfusion reactions and requires transfusion of blood for oxygen-carrying capacity should be transfused with

    A. Fresh Whole Blood
    B. Red Blood Cells
    C. Leukocyte-Poor Red Blood Cells
    D. Granulocytes obtained by cytopheresis

The answer is C. The cause of this patient's history of nonhemolytic febrile transfusion reactions probably is patient antibody reacting against donor leukocytes. To prevent these reactions one should remove leukocytes from blood transfused to the patient. Since the patient needs a transfusion for oxygen-carrying capacity (red blood cells), the component of choice is Leukocyte-Poor RBCs. (*Technical Manual of the American Association of Blood Banks*)

41. A patient experiences chills and fever, nausea, flushing, and lower back pain following the infusion of 350 ml of blood. To rule out quickly a transfusion reaction due to acute hemolysis, one should immediately

    A. Peform a direct antiglobulin test on the posttransfusion specimen.
    B. Culture the unit at 4°C, 22°C, and 32°C.
    C. Measure serum haptoglobin on pre- and postreaction samples.
    D. Repeat cross matches on pre- and postreaction specimens.

The answer is A. Although all of these measures help evaluate a hemolytic transfusion reaction, option A is the best and quickest to determine acute hemolysis. Other options are tests that can be done later, as determined necessary. (*Technical Manual of the American Association of Blood Banks*)

42. Which of the following antibodies is most often associated with delayed hemolytic transfusion reactions?

    A. A
    B. Jk^a
    C. Le^a
    D. M

The answer is B. Patients previously sensitized to Jk^a may have antibody titers drop to an undetectable level with time. Therefore, antibody screening will be negative and crossmatches will be compatible with these patients. However, antibody levels will rise to significant levels following transfusion with Jk^a-positive blood, causing a delayed transfusion reaction. (*Technical Manual of the American Association of Blood Banks*)

43. An *acute* hemolytic transfusion reaction most commonly is due to

    A. An ABO mismatch
    B. An Rh mismatch
    C. Circulatory overload
    D. Hepatitis (non-A, non-B)

The answer is A. Life-threatening hemolytic transfusion reactions are almost always due to ABO mismatch attributable to an identification error that results in the recipient receiving the wrong blood. (*Technical Manual of the American Association of Blood Banks*)

44. Which of the following matings has the potential to result in hemolytic disease of the newborn (HDN) (ABO and/or Rh)?

	Mother's Phenotype	Father's Phenotype
A.	O, DCcEe	O, DCe
B.	A, DCcEe, K-positive	O, DcE, K-negative
C.	B, dce	O, DCce
D.	AB, Dce, Jk^a-negative	A, dce, Jk^a-negative

The answer is C. HDN can occur when the fetus has antigens (inherited from its father) that the mother does not have. In option A there are no Rh antigens that are different from those of the mother. In option B there are no problems since the mother has all the Rh antigens as well as K; because the mother is A and the child is either A or O, ABO HDN cannot occur. In option C the Rh-negative woman could have an Rh-positive child, resulting in Rh HDN. In option D, the father has no Rh antigens that are different from those of the mother, so Rh HDN cannot occur; since the mother is AB, no ABO HDN can occur, and no sensitization to Jk^a can occur since the father is negative for this antigen. (Henry)

45. Laboratory studies of maternal and cord blood yield the following results:

Maternal Blood
O, $Rh_o(D)$-positive
Anti-c identified in serum

Cord Blood
A $Rh_o(D)$-positive
Direct antiglobulin test: 2 +
Anti-c identified in eluate

If exchange transfusion is required, the best choice of blood is

A. A-negative, c-positive
B. O-positive, c-negative
C. A-positive, c-positive
D. O-negative, c-negative

The answer is B. Donor blood of the baby's ABO group should be selected when known—*if* it is compatible with the mother's serum. In this instance, the O mother, with anti-A in her serum, would react with A cells if these were used. Thus, O red cells should be selected. Since the mother has anti-c in her serum, blood lacking c antigen should be used; thus, O cells, c-negative (e.g., CDe/CDe) should be used.
This example illustrates the possibility of hemolytic disease of the newborn due to an Rh antigen other than D. Since both mother and child are Rh-positive, Rh-positive blood (e.g., R^1R^1) may be used. (Henry)

46. A donor unit contains a warm-reacting (37°C) unexpected antibody. According to the AABB *Standards for Blood Banks and Transfusion Services,* what should be done with that unit?

A. It can be treated as any other unit for transfusion.
B. It should be used only for purposes other than red cell transfusion (e.g., plasma components).
C. It may be used only as frozen blood.
D. It should be used as Red Blood Cells, or the equivalent, with plasma removed.

The answer is D. The AABB *Standards for Blood Banks and Transfusion Services* suggests that donor units containing antibody that is reactive at 37°C should be processed into components that contain only minimal amounts of plasma. The antibody contained in the unit will be reduced in quantity, and on transfusion will become diluted within the recipient's body. (*Technical Manual of the American Association of Blood Banks*)

47. Whole blood collected in CPDA-1 (citrate-phosphate-dextrose with adenine) may be stored for up to

A. 48 hr
B. 21 days
C. 35 days
D. 42 days

The answer is C. CPDA-1 is "good" for 35 days, mainly because the additive adenine provides a substrate from which erythrocytes can synthesize ATP. (*Technical Manual of the American Association of Blood Banks*)

48. Which is the only solution that can be added to blood or components before or during transfusion?

   A. Normal saline
   B. Double-distilled water
   C. 10% heparin
   D. Lactated Ringer's solution

The answer is A. The AABB *Standards for Blood Banks and Transfusion Services* states that "only 9% sodium chloride may be added to blood or components." If distilled water were used, hemolysis of red cells would occur. Heparin might cause coagulation problems. Lactated Ringer's solution contains enough ionized calcium to overcome the anticoagulant effect and would allow clots to form. (*Technical Manual of the American Association of Blood Banks*)

49. The temperature of a refrigerator that contains stored blood should not exceed

   A. 4 C
   B. 6 C
   C. 8 C
   D. 10 C

The answer is B. According to the AABB, the temperature in a refrigerator used to store blood must be maintained between 1°C and 6°C. The refrigerator must also have a recording thermometer and an alarm system; often the alarm is set to trigger at 7°C. (*Technical Manual of the American Association of Blood Banks*)

50. Quality assurance of blood bank equipment does *not* include which of the following?

   A. Weekly calibration of centrifuges used in serologic testing
   B. Testing the temperature of heating blocks and water baths at a determined point on each day of use
   C. Periodic testing of the high and low activation temperatures of the blood bank alarm system
   D. Periodic checks of the volume of antiglobulin serum delivered by cell washers that automatically add antiglobulin serum

The answer is A. Options B, C, and D are required to check that the equipment is working well. The AABB recommends that quality control be performed for centrifuges, cell washers, water baths, heating blocks and incubators, Rh view boxes, and refrigerators and freezers. Centrifuges should be calibrated on receipt and following repairs and adjustments. (*Technical Manual of the American Association of Blood Banks*)

CLS Review Questions

1. Match the following definitions with the terms provided.

   Definitions
   1. Average strength of binding between antigens and antibodies
   2. Nonspecific attachment of substances to the surfaces of insoluble particles
   3. Use of reagents to remove certain antigens (or antibodies) from a mixture (e.g., to remove anti-E from a mixture of anti-C and anti-E)

   Terms
   a. Absorption
   b. Adsorption
   c. Avidity

   A. 1-a; 2-c; 3-b
   B. 1-c; 2-a; 3-b
   C. 1-c; 2-b; 3-a
   D. 1-b; 2-a; 3-c

The answer is C. Definitions are as follows:

Absorption: using reagents to remove unwanted antigens or antibodies from a mixture by serologic reaction (e.g., absorption-elution techniques to separate antibodies)

Adsorption: the nonspecific attachment of substances, such as proteins, to surfaces of red cells or inert particles (e.g., the adsorption of a drug onto the surface of a red blood cell, resulting in a positive direct antiglobulin test)

Avidity: the binding strength exhibited by antibodies of a given serum to a complex antigen (e.g., a highly avid serum is one that binds its homologous antigens tightly; highly avid serums tend to give larger "scores" to reactions that are graded). (Bryant; Roitt, Glossary)

2. "Immune" A and B alloantibodies differ from "natural" A and B alloantibodies in that the "immune" antibodies

   A. Are generally IgG
   B. Are unable to cross the placenta
   C. Can have their titer enhanced by incubation at cold temperature
   D. Cause direct agglutination at room temperature

The answer is A. The major differences between natural and immune alloantibodies are outlined below:

	Natural	Immune
Class	IgM	IgG
Ability to cross placenta	No	Yes
Optimal temperature of reactivity	$\leq 22°C$	37°C
Serologic characteristics	Usually cause direct agglutination	Usually require AHG for agglutination

(*Technical Manual of the American Association of Blood Banks*)

3. Which of the following is an example of a type I hypersensitivity reaction?

   A. Allergic reaction to grass pollen
   B. Systemic lupus erythematosus
   C. TB skin reaction
   D. Autoimmune hemolytic anemia

The answer is A. Coombs and Gell have described four types of hypersensitivity reactions. Type I reactions, also called anaphylactic reactions, occur within minutes and are mediated by IgE antibodies. These reactions involve the release of pharmacologic mediators from basophils and mast cells. In type II reactions, antibodies are directed against an individual's own red cells. Examples include autoimmune hemolytic anemias and thrombocytopenic purpura. Type III reactions involve the deposition of immune complexes in the tissues. Systemic lupus erythematosus and poststreptococcal glomerulonephritis are examples. In type IV hypersensitivity reactions, sensitized T cells release lymphokines following a secondary exposure to antigen. The TB skin reaction and contact dermatitis are examples. (Henry)

4. Interpret the Ouchterlony double diffusion reaction pattern seen below. Wells 1 and 2 contain antigen(s). Well 3 contains antibody(ies).

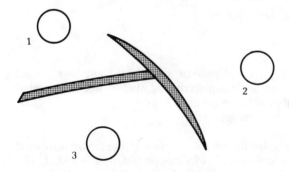

   A. Two patterns of nonidentity
   B. A pattern of partial identity
   C. Patterns of identity and nonidentity
   D. Two patterns of identity

The answer is B. In the classic Ouchterlony double diffusion test, two different solutions of antigens can react with one antiserum. If the solutions contain the same antigen, the proximal tips of their negative lines of precipitate will fuse, giving a line of identity (⌒). If they contain different antigens and the antigen contains preciptins to both, their lines of precipitate will cross, giving a reaction of nonidentity (✗). Partially related antigens will form intermediate reactions, as can be seen in this example. (Bellanti)

5. Which of the following fractions is elevated most often in multiple myeloma?

   A. Albumin
   B. Alpha (alpha$_1$ or alpha$_2$)
   C. Beta
   D. Gamma

The answer is D. Multiple myeloma is characterized as a disease of plasma cells, in which the plasma cells contain or secrete a single type of immunoglobulin (monoclonal). These may be of any of the immunoglobulin classes; of all patients with multiple myeloma, about 50% have IgG proteins and 25% have IgA proteins. Electrophoretic (or immunoelectrophoretic) analysis of patients with multiple myeloma often shows a characteristic peak of protein (the myeloma spike), seen most often in the gamma fraction. (Stites et al.)

6. The results below represent a viral hemagglutination inhibition test. The titer of the first tube is 1:10, and doubling dilutions are used thereafter. What interpretation of these results can be made?

Tube No.

1	2	3	4	5	6	7	8	9	10
1:10							Virus control	Serum control	RBC control
0	0	0	0	0	+	+	+	0	0

Key: + = agglutination; 0 = no agglutination.

The results are

   A. Invalid due to the virus control pattern and should not be reported
   B. Invalid due to the serum control pattern and should not be reported
   C. Valid; a titer of 1:160 should be reported
   D. Valid; a titer of 1:320 should be reported

The answer is C. For this hemagglutination inhibition test, the serum is diluted as 1:10, 1:20, 1:40, etc. A constant amount of virus preparation is added. The cells settle, and the pattern of sedimented cells is read. The end point is the highest dilution of serum that will *inhibit* hemagglutination by the virus. All controls are valid; the virus control (containing no serum) shows hemagglutination; the serum control (containing no virus) shows that the serum used had no antibodies to red blood cells; the red blood cell control contains only red blood cells and shows no spontaneous agglutination. The end point of the test is read at the highest dilution of serum that inhibits hemagglutination. This is tube 5, representing a 1:160 titer. (Stites et al.)

7. In some laboratories, one-dimensional electroimmunoassay may be used in addition to radial immunodiffusion. Which of the following is a characteristic of electroimmunoassay?

   A. It is a qualitative rather than quantitative test.
   B. It is performed in test tubes, like the Oudin test.
   C. Lines of identity and nonidentity can be distinguished easily.
   D. Antigen is moved by electrophoresis rather than diffusion.

The answer is D. One-dimensional electroimmunoassay, also known as rocket immunoelectrophoresis, is often used to quantitate proteins (e.g., immunoglobulins). It uses special electrophoresis equipment and plates of gel containing immobilized antibody. The pH of the gel medium is 8.6. Wells are cut in the gel, antigen added, moistened filter paper wicks added, and current applied. Antigen is pulled into the gel forming a rocket-shaped band of precipitate, in which the length of the rocket is proportional to the logarithm of the antigen concentration. (Stites et al.)

8. A 22-year-old man is seen in a clinic with an ulcerative lesion on his penis. The diagnosis of primary syphilis in this patient can best be established by

   A. FTA-ABS
   B. Testing for the presence of reagin
   C. Culturing the organism from the penis
   D. Dark-field examination of material from the ulcer

The answer is D. A positive dark-field examination is the only means of making an absolute diagnosis of primary syphilis. If the initial dark-field examination is negative, syphilis is not excluded. The lesion should be examined by dark-field microscopy on 2 successive days and additional serologic test obtained. (Henry)

9. Heterophile antibodies in infectious mononucleosis are

   A. Not of the Forssman type and not absorbed by suspensions of guinea pig kidney
   B. Not of the Forssman type and absorbed by suspensions of guinea pig kidney
   C. Of the Forssman type and not absorbed by suspensions of guinea pig kidney
   D. Of the Forssman type and absorbed by suspensions of guinea pig kidney

The answer is A. Heterophile antibodies of the Forssman type are characterized by reactions with (absorption by) suspensions of guinea pig kidney. The heterophile antibodies found in infectious mononucleosis are not of the Forssman type and are not absorbed by guinea pig kidney. (Henry)

10. The following results are seen in an antistreptolysin O (ASO) test on a 35-year-old man (red cell control–no lysis; streptolysin control–total hemolysis):

Tube No.	1	2	3	4	5	6	7	8	9
Positive control	No lysis	No lysis	No lysis	No lysis	Slight hemolysis	Total hemolysis	Total hemolysis	Total hemolysis	Total hemolysis
Patient	No lysis	No lysis	No lysis	No lysis	No lysis	No lysis	Slight hemolysis	Total hemolysis	Total hemolysis
Todd units	12	50	100	125	166	250	333	500	625

What is your conclusion based on these results?

A. The patient's ASO titer is within the normal range for an adult.
B. The patient's ASO titer is indicative of recent group A streptococcal infection.
C. The results are invalid, due to partial hemolysis in some tubes.
D. Results are invalid due to the control results.

The answer is B. Low ASO titers are seen in the majority of the population, but the "normal" level varies widely with age and geographic locale. Levels for preschool youngsters and mature adults are generally less than 100 Todd units, whereas school-age children, teenagers, college students, and members of the armed services have slightly higher levels (e.g., 166 Todd units). It is important to remember that a low titer may be normal and that regional and hospital norms exist.

Acute and convalescent ASO titers are desirable for good diagnostic workups. Significant elevations of titer, 250 Todd units or greater, are indicative of recent group A streptococcal infection. The control values are correct, and slight hemolysis can occur in some tubes (i.e., tubes that are between those showing no lysis and those showing total hemolysis). (Bryant)

11. In an ASO test, the streptolysin O control tube demonstrates no lysis. What might be the effect on the results of the test?

A. Falsely elevated values
B. No effect, since the end point is read as the highest dilution demonstrating hemolysis
C. No effect, since all tubes would be equally affected
D. Falsely decreased values

The answer is A. The principle of the ASO test is as follows: Streptolysin O causes the lysis of erythrocytes; in the presence of a neutralizing antibody (ASO), however, hemolysis of cells is inhibited. The end point of this test is read as the highest serum dilution showing no hemolysis. The absence of hemolysis in the streptolysin O control tube indicates inactivation of the reagent. Thus a falsely elevated value will be obtained, since the reagent streptolysin O is not effective in hemolyzing erythrocytes. (Rose et al.)

12. In rheumatic fever, damage to the heart appears to result from

    A. Streptococcal activation of forbidden clones
    B. Stimulation of delayed hypersensitivity response
    C. Antigenic similarity of myocardial tissue and group A streptococci
    D. Alteration of myocardial antigens by group A streptococci

The answer is C. In rheumatic fever, damage to the heart appears to be related to the patient's production of antibody against group A streptococcal antigens, which are similar to normal myocardial tissue antigens. The similarity of streptococcal and myocardial antigens appears to permit the antibodies against streptococcal antigens to cross-react with certain antigens of the patient's myocardial tissue. (Stites et al.)

13. The preferred procedure for measuring streptococcal antibodies formed during streptococcal pyoderma (streptococcal skin disease) is

    A. Anti-DNA
    B. Anti-DNase B
    C. Antirheumatoid factor
    D. Antistreptokinase

The answer is B. Although the ASO test has been used extensively to check for streptococcal infection, streptococcal deoxyribonuclease (also called streptodornase) has proved especially helpful in determining a serologic reaction to streptococcal pyoderma. Actually, group A streptococci produce four deoxyribonucleases—A, B, C, and D—of which DNase B is the most antigenically consistent. Several tests for anti-DNase B are available. Antibodies to DNase B rise later and remain elevated longer than antibodies to streptolysin O. Detection of anti-DNase B can be valuable in documenting a streptococcal infection in a patient with acute rheumatic fever or acute glomerulonephritis after an infection of either the throat or skin. (Rose et al.)

14. All of the following are characteristics of "cold agglutinins" *except*

    A. They react optimally at temperatures between 1° and 10°C.
    B. They can give a reversible reaction after warming.
    C. They are strongly reacting with cord cells.
    D. They agglutinate almost all adult human red blood cells, regardless of group.

The answer is C. Cold agglutinins are antibodies that are usually not clinically important. They tend to react best at about 5°C. Formerly, they were considered to be nonspecific. Because most are associated with anti-I, they react with most human adult red cells (at 1–10°C) but not cord cells, which are high in i antigen. The reaction is reversible on warming. (Stites et al.)

15. A titer is set up for rheumatoid factor. The following results are obtained for the positive control (Agg=agglutination; Neg=negative):

Tube No.	1	2	3	4	5	6	7	8	9	10
Positive control titer	1:10	1:20	1:40	1:80	1:160	1:320	1:640	1:1280	1:2560	Antigen control
Results	Agg	Agg	Agg	Agg	Agg	Agg	Agg	Neg	Neg	Neg

The patient's results are shown below:

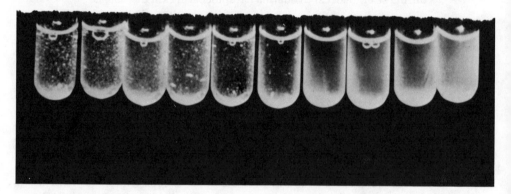

The results seen above are

A. Invalid and the patient's results should not be reported
B. Valid and the patient's results should be reported as a titer of 1:160
C. Valid and the patient's results should be reported as a titer of 1:320
D. Valid and the patient's results should be reported as a titer of 1:640

The answer is C. The positive control gives results that are correct, including the antigen control, which should show no agglutination. The end point for the patient is seen in tube 6 of the photograph, which indicates a titer of 1:320. (Henry)

16. The highest titers of antithyroglobulin antibodies are seen in

A. Addison's disease
B. Carcinoma of the thyroid
C. Graves' disease
D. Hashimoto's thyroiditis

The answer is D. Antithyroglobulin antibodies can be found in several disorders of the thyroid, as well as in some other autoimmune diseases. The titer of antibody is generally low, except in Hashimoto's thyroiditis. (Henry)

17. In Addison's disease, the most common autoantibody has specificity for

    A. Nuclear constituents
    B. Skeletal muscle
    C. The adrenal cortex
    D. Thyroid microsomes

The answer is C. Autoantibodies to adrenocortical cells are detected in up to 60% of persons with idiopathic Addison's disease. An indirect immunofluorescence test is usually used; the antibodies detected stain the cytoplasm of cells of the adrenal cortex. They are directed to antigen associated with the microsomes of these cells. (Henry)

18. Glomerulonephritis has been associated with systemic lupus erythematosus and serum sickness. In these instances one may consider this kidney condition to be caused by a(n)

    A. Autoimmune reaction
    B. Reaction caused by alloantibodies
    C. Delayed hypersensitivity (type IV) reaction
    D. Immediate hypersensitivity (type I) reaction

The answer is A. In this type of glomerulonephritis, autologous antibodies are complexed with nonglomerular antigens. These become trapped in the capillaries. (Henry)

19. A patient has signs and symptoms of gastroenteritis. The rapid slide test for one of the *Salmonella* H antigens is positive at a 1:80 dilution of serum. This result

    A. Should be confirmed by direct culture
    B. Is diagnostic of *Salmonella* gastroenteritis
    C. Would be significant if it represented a twofold increase in titer
    D. Should be confirmed with tests for cell-mediated immune responses to *Salmonella*

The answer is A. A titer of 1:80 on a screening test may or may not indicate *Salmonella* infection. Because interpretation is difficult, this reaction should be confirmed by direct culture of the infecting organism. The titer of 1:80 may also represent recent infection with other members of the Enterobacteriaceae family. A fourfold rise in titer of paired sera initially and several (e.g., 3) weeks later would be considered good evidence of infection. Tests for cell-mediated immune responses to *Salmonella* are not available. (Stites et al.)

20. Although the recovery and identification of fungi from clinical specimens is preferred when making a diagnosis of a fungal infection, this cannot always be done. Several serologic tests for fungi can be employed, one of which is for infection from *Histoplasma*. In this instance, serologic testing is most commonly performed by means of

    A. Direct agglutination of nonattenuated *Histoplasma capsulatum* yeast forms
    B. Precipitation in tubes
    C. Viral neutralization
    D. Complement fixation

The answer is D. Option A is eliminated because yeast forms of pathogenic organisms are not normally used in a direct agglutination test. Option B is eliminated because a precipitation reaction requires soluble antigen. Option C is incorrect because *Histoplasma* is not a virus. Option D is correct; this is the procedure most often used. (Henry)

21. In the 2-hr hemagglutination inhibition (HAI) test for human chorionic gonadotropin (hCG), in which ring = doughnut pattern and mat = uniform film pattern, a positive reaction is indicated by a

    A. Ring pattern in patient tube; smooth mat pattern in positive control tube
    B. Similar smooth mat patterns in both patient and positive control tubes
    C. Similar ring patterns in both patient and positive control tubes
    D. Mat pattern substantially larger in patient tube than in positive control tube

The answer is C. HAI is based on the observation that nonagglutinated red cells settle in a test tube to form a sharply demarcated ring or doughnut, whereas agglutinated red cells form a uniform film or mat at the bottom of a test tube. In the HAI procedure, anti-hCG serum and erythrocytes coated with hCG are incubated with patient urine. If hCG is present in the patient's urine, it will neutralize the antiserum; if hCG is absent, the antiserum is not affected. An unaffected antiserum will agglutinate the red cells, and a diffuse mat of cells forms, indicating a negative reaction. However, if the antiserum is neutralized by hCG in the urine, the red cells form a doughnut or ring pattern, indicating a positive result. (Henry)

22. In a quantitative pregnancy test, a titer of 1:1024 (e.g., 2×10^6 mIU/ml) is most suggestive of

    A. Threatened spontaneous abortion
    B. Normal pregnancy—sixth month
    C. Normal pregnancy—third month
    D. Hydatidiform mole

The answer is D. Because this titer is extremely high, we can eliminate options A and B which are associated with low levels of hCG. The third month of a normal pregnancy may show moderate levels of hCG (e.g., 100,000 mIU/ml), since the peak levels seem to occur 70 days following implantation. However, these levels of hCG are extremely high and are most indicative of hydatidiform mole, a trophoblastic tumor. (Henry, pp. 497–498)

23. The technique most widely used to determine the presence of the HLA-A and HLA-B antigens is

   A. Fluorescent antibody
   B. Mixed lymphocyte culture
   C. Differential agglutination
   D. Lymphocyte cytotoxicity

The answer is D. The most widely used method for HLA-A and HLA-B typing is the lymphocyte cytotoxicity assay. Antiserum to HLA antigens is added to the wells of microtiter plate; peripheral blood lymphocytes are added to each well and incubated; complement is added and incubated; and dye is added. Cells lysed by antiserum and complement take up the dye; cells unaffected by the antiserum remain unstained. The fluorescent antibody technique is not widely used, and mixed lymphocyte culture would not indicate antigen type (except for D). Differential agglutination is a fictitious distractor. (Henry)

24. A patient with antibodies directed against antigens of the HLA system may experience any of the following *except*

   A. Febrile reactions to blood transfusion
   B. Rejection of a renal transplant
   C. Poor response to platelet transfusion
   D. Increase in complement levels

The answer is D. Persons may develop antibodies to HLA antigens. For example, if a patient has lymphocytotoxic antibodies against donor cells, a kidney transplant can be expected to be rejected immediately. HLA antibodies are also crucial in bone marrow transplants. The patient transfused repeatedly with platelets may also build antibodies to HLA antigens. Leukocyte antibodies have been implicated in febrile transfusion reactions. Levels of complement do not increase as a result of antigenic stimulation. (*Technical Manual of the American Association of Blood Banks*)

25. Which of the following is found frequently in patients with liver cancer?

   A. Alpha-fetoprotein
   B. hCG
   C. Ferritin
   D. Antihyaluronidase

The answer is A. Cancer cells often shift backward from an adult to a fetal pathway of protein production. In this instance, one of the serologic indicators of liver cancer is alpha-fetoprotein (AFP). AFP is an $alpha_1$-globulin, similar to albumin. It is found in the yolk sac and early fetal liver and disappears in utero with maturity. However, it may reappear in liver cancer and other conditions, such as viral hepatitis, lung tumors, or pancreatic tumors. (Stites et al.)

26. Below are listed the results of a donor history:

   Traveled to an area considered endemic for malaria 18 months ago; has had no antimalarial drugs or symptoms of malaria

   Has seasonal hay fever; presently is asymptomatic

   Has not eaten for the past 12 hr

   Takes an occasional sleeping pill

   How many of these results exclude the person from giving blood for routine transfusion?

   A. None
   B. One
   C. Two
   D. Three

The answer is A. Although none of the conditions listed should exclude the donor, items concerning the hay fever, fasting, and sleeping pills warrant additional consideration. If the donor is taking aspirin or aspirin-containing medications, the blood should not be the only source of platelets for a patient. Because lack of eating often causes more donor reactions than usual, a light snack before donation is advisable. The occasional use of hypnotics often is acceptable, but it is advised in such instances that the donor's verbal approval to donate be documented on the donor record. (*Technical Manual of the American Association of Blood Banks*)

27. Which of the following gives all the possible phenotypes of offspring that could result from the mating of a group A person with a group B person?

   A. A and B only
   B. A and B and AB only
   C. A and B and O only
   D. A and B and AB and O

The answer is D. The phenotype A or B of the parents could be of the genotype AO or BO. Since one gene from each parent is passed to an offspring, any combination could result.

Example:

                    Parent 1
                     A   O
Parent 2   B | AB | BO | Offspring
            O | AO | OO | possibilities

(*Technical Manual of the American Association of Blood Banks*)

28. A patient whose blood is a subgroup of A gives the following red blood cell reactions:

Dolichos biflorus: negative
Anti-A: mixed-field agglutination
Anti-A,B: mixed-field agglutination

This patient has an anti-A_1. Most likely, the subgroup of A is

A. A_1
B, A_2
C. A_3
D. A_m

The answer is C. The mixed-field reactions with anti-A and anti-A,B are characteristic of the subgroup A_3. Occasionally, A_3 persons have anti-A_1 in their serum. (A_3 persons who are ABH secretors have both A and H substance in their saliva.) (*Technical Manual of the American Association of Blood Banks*)

29. The presence of anti-A_1 is usually detected by

A. The antibody screening cells procedure (indirect Coombs' test)
B. Reverse ABO grouping procedure
C. Red cell typing antisera
D. Use of A_2 cells

The answer is B. Anti-A_1 will react with the A_1 cells used in reverse typing. Anti-A_1 will not react with the O cells used for antibody screening. Since we are considering anti-A_1, other antisera (e.g., typing sera) will have no effect, and anti-A_1 will not be expected to react with A_2 cells. (*Technical Manual of the American Association of Blood Banks*)

30. Which of the following best reflects the discrepancy seen when a person demonstrates an "acquired B-like" phenomenon?

A. Forward typing appears to be B, but reverse groups like O.
B. Foward typing appears to be AB, but reverse groups like A.
C. Forward typing appears to be O, but reverse groups like B.
D. Forward typing appears to be B, but reverse groups like AB.

The answer is B. Some group A people, such as those with carcinoma of the colon, massive infection with gram-negative organisms, or intestinal obstruction have been found to "acquire" a B-like antigen. Gerbal suggested that "acquired B" may result from the action of bacterial deacetylase, which converts N-acetyl-galactosamine to N-galactosamine, which is similar to galactose (the primary determinant of B). Interestingly, the patient's own natural anti-B does not react with the B-like antigen on his or her own cells, whereas most other anti-Bs react with the patient cells. (*Technical Manual of the American Association of Blood Banks*)

31. Select the most likely cause for the ABO forward and reverse reactions given below:

Cell grouping			Serum grouping			
Anti-A	Anti-B	Anti-A,B	A cells	B cells	O cells	Autocontrol
4+	0	4+	0	0	0	0

   A. Polyagglutinable cells
   B. Immunodeficiency
   C. Acquired A-like antigen
   D. A subgroup

The answer is B. The strong reactions in the forward grouping indicate a group A person. However, no agglutination is seen in the reverse grouping, in which the serum of a group A person possessing anti-B should react with B cells. One would not expect reactions with A cells or O cells. The autocontrol is negative, ruling out an autoantibody. The lack of agglutination in any of the serum groupings or with the autocontrol causes one to suspect an immunodeficiency, in which the person does not produce antibodies demonstrable at 22°C (room temperature). (*Technical Manual of the American Association of Blood Banks*)

32. The following results are obtained when a patient's saliva is tested for ABH secretor status:

(Saliva + anti-A) + A cells: 4+
(Saliva + anti-B) + B cells: 0
(Saliva + anti-H) + O cells: 1+

   It would be correct to assume that the patient's ABO blood group and secretor status are

   A. A, secretor
   B. A, nonsecretor
   C. B, nonsecretor
   D. B, secretor

The answer is D. In the secretor test, *inhibition* of specific agglutination indicates the presence of blood group substances in saliva. Thus, *no agglutination* indicates a positive result for the secretion of A, B, or H substances. The patient presented is a secretor, because no reaction occurs when B cells are added to the tube. B substance in the saliva reacts with anti-B. When B cells are added, there is no anti-B to react with them, and no agglutination is seen. The substances in saliva and on red cells are the same, although in different forms for solubility. People who have B substance in their secretions should also have B substance on their red cells. (*Technical Manual of the American Association of Blood Banks*)

33. The symbol cDE of the Fisher-Race system corresponds to the Wiener symbol

   A. R^o
   B. R^1
   C. R^2
   D. R^z

The answer is C. The following correspondences can be made:

Wiener Terminology		Fisher-Race Terminology	
Allelle	Major Antigenic Specificities	Gene Combination	Antigenic Specificities
R^1	Rh_o,rh',hr''	CDe	C,D,e
r	hr',hr''	cde	c,e
R^2	Rh_o,hr',rh''	cDE	c,D,E
R^o	Rh_o,hr',hr''	cDe	c,D,e
r'	rh',hr''	Cde	C,e
r''	hr',rh''	cdE	c,E
R^z	Rh_o,rh',rh''	CDE	C,D,E
r^y	rh',rh''	CdE	C,E

Source: Adapted from *Technical Manual of the American Association of Blood Banks* (9th ed.). Philadelphia: Lippincott, 1985, p. 130.

34. If a patient has an anti-c antibody, which of the following units of blood may he or she receive without an expected reaction due to this antibody?

   A. R^1R^2
   B. R^1R^1
   C. R^1r
   D. rr

The answer is B. A person who has anti-c should receive blood that does not contain corresponding antigens. R^1R^2 = CDe/cDE; R^1R^1 = CDe/CDe; R^1r = CDe/cde; and rr = cde/cde. Only R^1R^1 contains C/C and not c; therefore, it is the unit of choice to prevent antigen-antibody reactions. (*Technical Manual of the American Association of Blood Banks*)

35. A clinical laboratory scientist is asked to offer expert opinion in a paternity suit. All typings are done in duplicate, with appropriate controls. Given the following information, what conclusions can be drawn?

Mother   A, MN
Baby   O, NN
Alleged father O, MN

A. The typing procedures are probably in error.
B. Paternity is not excluded.
C. Paternity is excluded based on ABO results.
D. Paternity is excluded based on MN results.

The answer is B. The baby is O and could be the result of an AO mother and an OO father; ABO grouping does not exclude the alleged father. The baby is NN, a possibility from an MN mother and an MN father. Based on these results, the alleged father could be the father of the child. (Henry)

36. A drug that can cause a positive direct antiglobulin result by the "drug-adsorption" mechanism is

A. Methyldopa
B. Penicillin
C. Phenacetin
D. Quinidine

The answer is B. With penicillin (and cephalosporin) therapy, the patient may develop an antidrug antibody that reacts with the drug adsorbed onto the patient's red cells. The end result is a drug-coated red blood cell sensitized with IgG, detected as a positive direct antiglobulin result. (*Technical Manual of the American Association of Blood Banks*)

37. The blood bank receives an order of 4 units of blood for a surgical patient. Blood typing results are as follows:

Cell grouping
Anti-A: no agglutination
Anti-B: agglutination
Anti-A,B: agglutination
Anti-Rh$_o$ (D) through D^u testing: no agglutination
Autocontrol: no agglutination

Serum grouping
A cells: agglutination
B cells: agglutination

The next step required to resolve this problem is to

A. Draw a new blood sample from the patient to repeat all test procedures.
B. Set up a cell panel to identify the antibody causing the typing problem.
C. Test the patient's serum with A$_2$ cells and the patient's red cells with anti-A$_1$ lectin.
D. Repeat the ABO antigen typing using 3X washed saline-suspended cells.

The answer is B. There is a discrepancy in the ABO grouping. The patient appears to be a B according to forward typing reactions; however, the serum has reactions with both A and B cells. Since the D^u testing results show no agglutination, the problem is most likely due to the presence of an unexpected antibody that is reacting with the B cells. In this instance, performing a panel to identify this antibody is most appropriate. (*Technical Manual of the American Association of Blood Banks*)

38. Reagent red cells used in routine procedures to detect unexpected antibodies (indirect antiglobulin tests) do *not* detect which of the following alloantibodies?

   A. Anti-E
   B. Anti-H
   C. Anti-B
   D. Antibodies to high-frequency antigens

The answer is C. Reagent red cells are group O because they contain most of the antigens (other than A and B) to which antibodies may be produced. The fact that the cells are group O also rules out antibodies such as anti-A and anti-B. However, unexpected antibodies such as anti-H would be detected on O cells since O cells are high in H substance. Antibodies to high-frequency antigens would also be detected, since the O cells would contain these antigens. (*Technical Manual of the American Association of Blood Banks*)

39. Thomas Hanson, aged 53 years, is scheduled for open heart surgery. He is O-positive. Mr. Hanson has a previous history of transfusion, including 5 units of whole blood transfused in 1974. His phenotype is O, CDe. Results of the antibody screening test indicate an unexpected antibody. A cell panel is used to help identify the antibody. The results of the panel on page 104 suggest that the unexpected antibody is most likely

   A. Anti-K
   B. Anti-Do^a
   C. Anti-c
   D. Anti-E

The answer is C. One can eliminate anti-D, C, e, M, S, s, P$_1$, k, Fy^b, Jk^a, Jk^b, Le^b, and Xg^a by cell 5, for which no reactions are seen. This leaves the possibility of anti-E, c, N, K, Fy^a, Le^a, Do^a, and Sd^a. From these remaining, cell 7 eliminates anti-N, K, Fy^a, Le^a, Do^a, and Sd^a, leaving the possibilities of anti-E and anti-c. The pattern of reaction is identical to that of anti-c, which shows positive reactions with the c-positive cells and no reaction with the c-negative cells. Thus anti-c is the most logical antibody, although one must not rule out anti-E, which might be masked by the presence of anti-c. Since 17% of donors have the cDE (R^2) gene complex, this man, who has neither antigen, could produce anti-c and anti-E. Anti-c also reacts optimally at 37°C and with AHG. It is not a cold-reacting antibody as the panel results indicate. (*Technical Manual of the American Association of Blood Banks*)

Cell	D	C	E	c	e	M	N	S	s	P₁	K	k	Fyᵃ	Fyᵇ	Jkᵃ	Jkᵇ	Leᵃ	Leᵇ	Xgᵃ	Doᵃ	Sdᵃ	Saline RT	Albumin IS	Albumin 37°C	AHG	Papain IS	Papain 37°C
1. Ror	+	0	0	+	+	+	0	0	+	+	0	+	+	0	0	+	0	0	0	+	0	0	0	1+	3+	2+	4+
2. r'r Bg	0	+	0	+	+	+	+	+	0	0	0	+	+	+	0	+	0	+	+	+	+	0	0	0	2+	+	4+
3. r'r	0	0	0	+	+	0	+	+	+	0	0	+	0	+	+	0	0	0	0	+	++	0	0	1+	3+	2+	4+
4. rr	0	0	0	+	+	+	+	+	+	+	0	+	0	+	+	+	w+	+	0	0	0	0	0	1+	3+	2+	4+
5. RʷR¹	+	0	0	0	+	+	0	+	+	++	0	+	0	+	+	+	0	+	+	+	0	0	0	0	0	0	0
6. R²R² Coᵇ	+	+	+	0	0	+	+	0	+	+	0	+	+	+	0	+	+	+	+	+	++	0	0	1+	3+	2+	4+
7. R¹R¹ chidow+ Kk	+	+	0	0	+	+	+	+	+	+	+	+	+	+	0	+	+	0	+	+	+	0	0	0	0	0	0
8. rr KK	0	0	0	+	+	+	0	+	+	+	+	0	+	0	+	0	0	0	0	++	++	0	0	1+	3+	2+	4+
9. R²R² Ykᵃ⁻	+	+	+	+	0	+	+	+	+	+	0	+	0	+	+	+	+	0	+	+	0	0	0	1+	3+	2+	4+

RT = room temperature; IS = initial spin; AHG = antihuman globulin.

40. A patient has imcompatibile crossmatches and a positive antibody screen in the antiglobulin phase. The patient's serum is tested against a panel of reagent red blood cells. Reactions are shown in the panel on page 106.

What are the most probable antibodies?

A. Anti-S and k
B. Anti-S and Fy^a
C. Anti-K and Fy^a
D. Anti-S and K and Fy^a

The answer is C. The choice of antibodies using this panel includes anti-D, C, E, c, e, M, N, S, s, Le^a, Le^b, P$_1$, K, k, Fy^a, Fy^b, Jk^a, and Jk^b. No reaction is seen in the autocontrol tube, indicating that an autoimmune antibody is not present. The antibodies must be alloantibodies.

Cells 1, 4, 7, and 8 give negative reactions, so those antibodies that would have given positive reactions with the antigens on the cells can be eliminated. This leaves the possibility of anti-S, K, and Fy^a. These three antibodies have optimal reactivity in the antiglobulin test (AGT). None of the antibodies is reactive in saline at room temperature. Reactions of + and 2+ are recorded in low ionic strength salt solutions (LISS) at 37°C.

The reactions seen coincide with the pattern shown for anti-K. K antigen is present on cells 2, 6, and 9 (LISS AGT brings stronger reactions with these cells); additional reaction is seen with cells 3, 5, and 10. Cells 3, 5, 6, and 10 also fit the pattern of Fy^a. Ficin treatment destroys Duffy reactions. Following ficin treatment, only cells 2, 6, and 9 react (corresponding to anti-K), indicating that Fy^a has been removed by the ficin treatment.

K is present in the homozygous form (KK) on cells 6 and 9 and in the heterozygous form (Kk) on cell 2. The reactions correspond to this, with 4+ reactions seen with cells 6 and 9 and a 3+ reaction with cell 2.

The most logical antibodies identified by this panel are anti-K and anti-Fy^a. However, anti-S cannot be totally ruled out because it might be masked by the presence of the other two antibodies. (*Technical Manual of the American Association of Blood Banks*)

41. A donor gives incompatible major crossmatches in the antiglobulin phase with seven of seven different recipients of the same ABO and Rh type. Based on these results, the donor might be expected to be positive on

A. Direct antiglobulin test
B. Indirect antiglobulin test
C. Anti-I
C. k antigen typing

The answer is A. The major crossmatch uses recipient serum and donor cells. Therefore something on this donor's cells must be reacting with all recipient sera. The indirect antiglobulin test (option B) is eliminated since donor serum (not cells) is tested in that procedure. Option C is eliminated by similar reason-

Cell No.	D	C	E	c	e	M	N	S	s	Le^a	Le^b	P_1	K	k	Fy^a	Fy^b	Jk^a	Jk^b	Saline RT	LISS 37°	LISS AGT	Ficin 37°C	Ficin AGT
1	+	0	0	+	+	0	+	0	+	+	0	+	0	+	0	+	+	0	0	0	0	0	0
2	+	0	0	+	+	+	+	+	+	0	+	0	+	+	0	0	+	+	0	+	3+	+	3+
3	+	+	0	0	+	+	+	+	0	0	0	+	0	+	+	+	+	+	0	0	1+	0	0
4	+	+	0	+	0	0	+	0	+	+	0	+	0	+	0	+	0	+	0	0	0	0	0
5	0	0	+	+	+	0	0	0	+	+	0	+	0	+	+	0	0	+	0	2+	2+	2+	4+
6	0	0	0	+	+	0	+	0	+	0	+	c	+	0	0	0	0	0	0	0	4+	0	0
7	0	0	0	+	+	+	0	+	+	0	+	0	0	+	0	+	+	0	0	0	0	0	0
8	0	0	0	+	+	0	+	+	0	0	0	+	0	0	0	+	+	+	0	2+	4+	2+	4+
9	0	0	0	+	+	+	0	+	+	+	0	+	+	+	+	+	+	+	0	0	1+	0	0
10	0	0	0	+	+	+	+	/	/	0	+	+	0	/	/	/	/	/	0	±	2+	±	2+
11 Cord	/	/	/	/	/	/	/	/	/	0	/	/	0	/	/	/	/	0	0	/	/	/	/
Auto	+	+	0	+	+	+	0	+	+	+	+	+	+	+	0	+	+	0	0	0	0	0	0

Key: RT = room temperature; LISS = low ionic strength salt solution; AGT = antiglobulin test.

ing since Anti-I is a serum antibody. Option D is eliminated because although most persons do have the k antigen, rarely do recipients have anti-k; in this instance, all seven would have had to have anti-k. The most likely choice would be an unexpected antibody coating the red cells. Unexpected antibodies coating donor cells would give a positive reaction in the antiglobulin phase of the crossmatch. (*Technical Manual of the American Association of Blood Banks*)

42. A patient has a positive autologous control on immediate spin. All tests done at 37°C and with AHG are negative. The antibody is identified as anti-I. It is learned that the patient received several units of blood within the past month at another institution. What is the procedure of choice to obtain compatible blood now?

   A. Absorb the patient's serum with the donor's cells at 4°C.
   B. Absorb the patient's serum with the patient's cells at 4°C.
   C. Perform all tests at 37°C and convert to the antiglobulin phase.
   D. Perform warm autoabsorptions with the patient's cells and the patient's serum.

The answer is C. One should not absorb patient's serum with the donor's cells (option A). Since the patient history includes recent transfusion, autoabsorption (options B and D) would not be appropriate. Alloantibodies might be absorbed onto transfused cells in the patient's blood sample. Therefore, option C gives the procedure of choice. (*Technical Manual of the American Association of Blood Banks*)

43. For which of the following blood components is a crossmatch *required* before transfusion?

   A. Platelet Concentrate
   B. Single-Donor Fresh Frozen Plasma
   C. Single-Donor Cryoprecipitate
   D. Granulocyte Concentrate

The answer is D. Single-Donor Plasma, Single-Donor Fresh Frozen Plasma, Single-Donor Cryoprecipitate, and Platelet Concentrate may be transfused without a compatibility test (crossmatch). In contrast, red-cell compatibility testing must be performed before transfusion of Granulocyte Concentrate. (*Standards for Blood Banks and Transfusion Services*)

44. A 44-year-old woman has a hemoglobin level of 6.1 g/dl. Leukocyte and platelet counts are within normal limits. The patient is group O, $Rh_o(D)$-negative, with no unexpected blood group antibodies detected in her serum. Crossmatches are compatible. However, 15 minutes after the first transfusion is started, she experiences a sudden anaphylactic reaction, including difficulty in breathing and hives. Subsequent units of transfused Washed

Red Cells are tolerated well. The most probable explanation for these findings is that the

A. Patient has antibodies against IgM.
B. Patient has antibodies against IgA.
C. Donor has IgG antibodies.
D. Patient has antiplatelet antibodies.

The answer is B. These signs and symptoms are most characteristic of an allergic reaction, of which urticaria (hives) is the most common sign. IgA-deficient patients who have developed Anti-IgA may experience anaphylactic reactions. The reactions occur after the infusion of a small amount of blood or plasma and are characterized by coughing, respiratory distress, nausea, and shock.

Antihistamines such as diphenhydramine (Benadryl) are effective in reducing the incidence of allergic reactions. However, using Washed Red Cells (which have IgA removed) has proved even more effective in preventing an allergic reaction. (*Technical Manual of the American Association of Blood Banks*)

45. Rh sensitization is *least* likely to occur in a mating of an Rh-negative woman and an Rh-positive man when their blood groups are

A. Mother A; father O
B. Mother B; father A
C. Mother O; father A
D. Mother AB; father O

The answer is C. ABO incompatibility between mother and father tends to protect the mother from Rh immunization. If a mother is group O and her fetus is group A or B, maternal anti-A, anti-B, and anti-A,B will sensitize fetal red cells that enter the material bloodstream. These red cells are more likely to be removed from the maternal bloodstream before immunization can occur. (*Technical Manual of the American Association of Blood Banks*)

46. In which of the following situations would the administration of Rh immune globulin (RhIG) *not* be indicated?

	Mother	Newborn
A.	r″r; no antibody detected	R_or; direct antiglobulin test positive
B.	rr; no antibody detected	R_1r; direct antiglobulin test negative
C.	rr; with anti-E	R_1r; direct antiglobulin test positive
D.	r″r; with anti-D	R_2r; direct antiglobulin test positive

The answer is D. Administration of RhIG prevents the formation of anti-D in a mother. If the mother has been immunized to the D antigen, however, and has produced anti-D, RhIG would not have beneficial effects. If anti-D is detected in maternal serum, however, the laboratory clinician must determine whether the patient received RhIG during pregnancy. If so, the patient should receive additional immunoprophylaxis after delivery, because the anti-D that is detected in the antibody screening procedure indicates the presence of RhIG but does not indicate immunization to the D antigen. (*Technical Manual of the American Association of Blood Banks*)

47. A woman is diagnosed as having immune hemolytic anemia (IHA). Her direct antiglobulin test is positive, but an indirect antiglobulin test is negative. Absorption-elution techniques are employed to help identify the causative antibody. The eluate gives the following agglutination patterns with these O cells:

cDE/cDE: ±
cdE/cDE: ±
cde/cde: 4+
cDE/cde: 2+
CDe/cDE: 2+

From these results, specificity of the antibody appears to be

A. Anti-C
B. Anti-E
C. Anti-c
D. Anti-e

The answer is D. In this situation, the antibodies that could cause IHA are assumed to be anti-C, anti-D, anti-E, anti-c, or anti-e. A spectrum of reactivities from ± to 4+ is observed, indicating multiple antibodies and/or a "dosing" antibody. If we consider only the 2+ and 4+ reactions for the moment, the possibility of the antibody being anti-c, anti-D, or anti-E is unlikely since only ± results were obtained with cells cDE/cDE and cdE/cDE. Anti-C is eliminated because a 2+ reaction is seen with cell cDE/cde.

In contrast, cell cde/cde contains e in the homozygous form, and a 4+ reaction is seen. In addition, 2+ reactions are seen in cells cDE/cde and CDe/cDE, in which e is the heterozygous form, indicating a dosage effect in the reactions obtained. Therefore, anti-e is the most logical antibody. Additional resolution of the ± reactions may be indicated depending on the policies of the individual blood banking facility regarding the possible clinical importance of such reactions. (*Technical Manual of the American Association of Blood Banks*)

48. A patient with cold agglutinin syndrome is found to have a positive direct antiglobulin test (DAT). Which of the following proteins is most likely to be the cause of the positive DAT?

A. C3d
B. C4d
C. IgG
D. IgM

The answer is A. The cold agglutinin syndrome is one of the autoimmune hemolytic anemias and is associated with cold-reacting antibodies. In cold agglutinin syndrome, it is the anti-C3d in AHG that causes the positive direct antiglobulin test. (*Technical Manual of the American Association of Blood Banks*)

49. The following phenotype frequencies are noted:

JK (a − b +): 20%   Le (a + b −): 22%
Jk (a + b −): 28%   Le (a − b +): 72%
Jk (a + b +): 52%   Le (a − b −): 6%

If donors were ABO- and Rh-specific with a recipient, it would be *easiest* to find compatible blood if the recipient's unexpected antibody were

A. Anti-Jk^a
B. Anti-Jk^b
C. Anti-Le^a
D. Anti-Le^b

The answer is C. According to the above statistics, these antigens are present in the following percentages:

Jk^a: 80% of the population—includes those who are Jk(a + b −) and Jk(a + b +) Jk(a + b +)
Jk^b: 72% of the population—includes those who are Jk(a − b +) and Jk(a + b +)
Le^a: 22% of the population—includes those who are Le(a + b −)
Le^b: 72% of the population—includes only those who are Le(a − b +)

One wishes to obtain the lowest percentage (most infrequently found) if an unexpected antibody is found. In this instance—if anti-Le^a were present—only 22% of the population has the corresponding Le^a antigen, which would give an incompatible crossmatch. (*Technical Manual of the American Association of Blood Banks*)

50. Blood typing of serum to detect *rare* antigens should follow quality control procedures. Recommended quality control includes

A. Titering rare antisera on receipt
B. Checking the rare antisera reactivity daily to detect possible deterioration
C. Testing rare antisera at the time they are used
D. Using cells homozygous for the antigen in question as the positive control

The answer is C. The AABB recommends that commonly used antisera (e.g., anti-A, anti-B) be tested each day before the day's tests are begun. Antisera that are not used frequently should be tested with control cells at the time they are being used. (To test them daily might exhaust the supply.)

The AABB recommends that monitoring antisera potency be done with weakly reactive antigen (i.e., from cells heterozygous for the antigenic determinant). (*Technical Manual of the American Association of Blood Banks*)

References

Bellanti, J.A. *Immunology III*. Philadelphia: Saunders, 1985.

Bryant, N.J. *Laboratory Immunology and Serology*. (2nd ed.) Philadelphia: Saunders, 1986.

Gerbal, A., Maslet, C., Salmon, C. Immunological aspects of the acquired B antigen. *Vox Sang.* 28: 398–403, 1975.

Henry, J.B. (Ed.) *Clinical Diagnosis and Management by Laboratory Methods* (17th ed.). Philadelphia: Saunders, 1984.

Issitt, P.D. *Applied Blood Group Serology*. (3rd ed.). Miami, FL: Montgomery Scientific Disciplines, 1985.

Pittiglio, D.H. *Modern Blood Banking and Transfusion Practices*. Philadelphia: Davis, 1983.

Roitt, I. *Essential Immunology* (6th ed.). Oxford, Blackwell, 1988.

Rose, N.R., Friedman, H., and Fahey J.L. (Eds.). *Manual of Clinical Immunology* (3rd ed.). Washington, D.C.: American Society for Microbiology, 1986.

Standards for Blood Banks and Transfusion Services (12th ed.). Arlington, Va.: American Association of Blood Banks, 1987.

Stites, D.P., Stobo, J.D., and Wells, J.V. (Eds.). *Basic and Clinical Immunology* (6th ed.). Norwalk, Conn.: Appleton & Lange, 1987.

Widmann F.K. (Ed.). *Technical Manual of the American Association of Blood Banks* (9th ed.). Philadelphia: Lippincott, 1985.

Microbiology

Section Editors
Holly K. Hall, M.A.
Elizabeth B. Sawyer, B.S.

Contributors
Ann C. Albers, M.S.
J. Suzanne Ames, M.S.
Barbara A. Atkinson, M.A.
Janice Babcock, M.A.
Clare C. Bailey, Ph.D.
John S. Baker, M.S.
David G. Bobey, M.S.
Eileen Broberg, M.S.
Shirley Carreiro, M.S.
Louis B. Caruara, M.S.
Edna R. Coleman, M.S.
Suzanne Conner, M.A.
Barbara Cretini, M.Ed.
William B. Davis, Ph.D.
Mary Ann Fiene, M.S.
Fran Fisher, M.Ed.
Cynthia L. Fuller
John P. Garcia, Ph.D.
Lynne S. Garcia, M.A.
Diane Garza, M.S.
Pamela Huber
Jane Hudson, M.S.
Linda Jeff, M.A.
Wendy Kiehn, M.S.
Lynn A. LaBounty, Ph.D.
Royce Lairscey, M.S.
Lillian V. Lee
Frederick J. Marsik, Ph.D.
Jacquelyn E. McConnell, M.A.T.
Lee Anne McGonagle
Shirley McManigal, Ph.D.
D. E. Montefolka, Ed.D.
Susan D. Page, M.S.
Syed M. H. Qadri, Ph.D.
Susan M. Roman, M.S.C.
John P. Seabolt, M.S.
Martha E. Singer, Ph.D.
Romeo L. Sobrepena
H. M. Sottnek, Ph.D.

CLT Review Questions

1. Which of the following characteristics is *not* used to isolate or identify *Staphylococcus aureus*?

   A. Hemolysis on sheep blood agar
   B. Fermentation of mannitol
   C. Positive catalase test
   D. Positive coagulase test

The answer is A. S. *aureus*, which is the most important pathogenic staphylococcus, generally ferments mannitol and produces catalase and coagulase enzymes. Mannitol salt agar is a selective and differential agar used for the primary isolation of staphylococci. Even though S. *aureus* ferments mannitol to produce acid in the medium surrounding the colonies, this ability is shared by other staphylococci. Definitive identification of S. *aureus* usually involves characterization of the isolate as a catalase-positive, gram-positive coccus that is coagulase-positive. Hemolysis on sheep blood agar is a variable characteristic among the staphylococci that does not contribute to the isolation or identification of S. *aureus*. (Lennette et al.)

2. To differentiate between a coagulase-negative *Staphylococcus* species and a *Micrococcus* species, which of the following tests should be set up?

   A. Anaerobic acid production from glucose
   B. Catalase
   C. Novobiocin susceptibility
   D. Trehalose utilization

The answer is A. Differentiation between staphylococci and micrococci can be made using glucose fermentation media. Staphylococci produce acid from glucose anaerobically, whereas micrococci that can produce acid from glucose do so aerobically only. All members of the family Micrococcaceae are catalase-positive. Novobiocin susceptibility differentiates *Staphylococcus saprophyticus* from other coagulase-negative staphylococci. Trehalose utilization can be used to differentiate *Staphylococcus epidermidis* from other coagulase-negative staphylococci. (Lennette et al.)

3. A pustule drainage submitted for culture is plated onto primary media. After an 18-hr incubation, the sheep blood agar plate reveals a predominance of beta-hemolytic, white, porcelainlike colonies. Gram stain shows gram-positive cocci that are catalase-positive. The most appropriate test for additional identification of the isolate is

   A. Bacitracin
   B. Bile esculin
   C. Bile solubility
   D. Coagulase

The answer is D. Facultatively anaerobic gram-positive cocci that are beta-hemolytic on sheep blood agar can presumptively be considered to be of the Micrococcaceae or Streptococcaceae family. Most members of the Micrococcaceae family are strongly catalase-positive, whereas the Streptococcaceae are catalase-negative or weakly positive. The coagulase test will definitively identify *Staphylococcus aureus*, the most likely causative agent from this specimen source. Bacitracin, bile esculin, and bile solubility are tests used in the identification of streptococci that are ruled out by a positive catalase result. (Finegold et al.)

4. A 43-year-old female patient complains of a very sore throat. The throat swab that is submitted for routine culture grows a variety of diphtheroids; alpha- beta-, and nonhemolytic streptococci; staphylococci and neisseriae. The next step is to

   A. Report it as normal throat flora.
   B. Ask for a repeat collection to get a better specimen.
   C. Identify the beta-hemolytic streptococcus species.
   D. Identify the *Neisseria* species.

The answer is C. Routine throat cultures on persons over approximately 10 years of age are taken primarily to detect the presence of *Streptococcus pyogenes*. Any amount of group A, beta-hemolytic streptococci is considered pathogenic and of concern because of the possibility of subsequent rheumatic fever or acute glomerular nephritis. In this patient, therefore, the beta-hemolytic streptococcus species should be identified. All the other organisms enumerated in this specimen may be encountered in the normal oropharyngeal flora, including non-group A, beta-hemolytic streptococci. (Finegold et al.)

5. A nasopharyngeal culture grows a predominance of a beta-hemolytic colony-type on sheep blood agar at 18 hr. The isolate is susceptible to 0.04 unit of bacitracin. The most likely identification is beta-hemolytic streptococcus,

   A. Group A
   B. Group B
   C. Group D
   D. Not group A, B, or D

The answer is A. *Streptococcus pyogenes* is a probable etiologic agent of pharyngitis. This isolate is presumptively identified as beta-hemolytic streptococcus, group A, by demonstration of susceptibility to bacitracin. Group A streptococci are also bile esculin–negative and hippurate hydrolysis–negative. Group B streptococci hydrolyze hippurate. Group D streptococci hydrolyze esculin in the presence of 40% bile. Other beta-hemolytic streptococci that are not in group A, B, or D are generally resistant to bacitracin and negative to the other reactions given in this problem. (Finegold et al.)

6. Which of the following characteristics is *not* consistent with *Streptococcus pneumoniae?*

   A. Alpha hemolysis on sheep blood agar
   B. Bile solubility—positive
   C. Gram-positive, oval-shaped cocci in pairs
   D. Positive catalase test

The answer is D. *S. pneumoniae* is a gram-positive, oval, or lancet-shaped coccus that is seen microscopically in pairs and chains. On sheep blood agar, colonies produce alpha hemolysis. Definitive identification requires a negative catalase test to differentiate it from *Aerococcus viridans* and either a bile solubility test or susceptibility to ethylhydrocupreine hydrochloride (optochin) to differentiate it from viridans streptococci. (Lennette et al.)

7. *Neisseria* species can be identified and differentiated by

   A. Bile esculin hydrolysis
   B. Carbohydrate utilization
   C. Nitrate test
   D. Oxidase test

The answer is B. Members of the genus *Neisseria* are identified by demonstrating acid production from the degradation of carbohydrates. The standard basal medium is cystine trypticase agar (CTA) into which 1% filtered sterilized carbohydrate is added. Conventional carbohydrate testing includes the utilization of glucose, lactose, maltose, sucrose, and fructose. Nitrate reduction differentiates *Branhamella catarrhalis* from members of the genus *Neisseria*. Since all *Neisseria* are oxidase-positive, the oxidase test is not useful in their differentiation. Bile esculin hydrolysis is not used for testing this group of bacteria (Lennette et al.)

8. A small gram-positive rod that causes neonatal meningitis and septicemia is

   A. *Escherichia coli*
   B. *Corynebacterium diphtheriae*
   C. *Listeria monocytogenes*
   D. *Streptococcus agalactiae*

The answer is C. *L. monocytogenes* is a small gram-positive rod that causes meningitis and septicemia in neonates, elderly, and immunocompromised patients. *E. coli* is a gram-negative rod. *C. diphtheriae* is a small gram-positive rod that can cause diphtheria in unimmunized hosts. *S. agalactiae* is a gram-positive coccus. (Lennette et al.)

9. The X and V factors required for growth of *Haemophilus influenzae* are contained in

   A. Brain heart infusion broth
   B. Chocolate agar

C. Sheep blood agar
D. Thioglycollate broth

The answer is B. Chocolate agar is enriched with hemin (or X factor) and NAD coenzyme (or V factor). Among the more fastidious organisms, both *Haemophilus* and *Neisseria* species will grow on chocolate agar (Lennette et al.)

10. On a sheep blood agar plate, *Haemophilus influenzae* satellites around colonies of

A. Diphthenoids
B. *Streptococcus pyogenes*
C. *Haemophilus parainfluenzae*
D. *Staphylococcus aureus*

The answer is D. *H. influenzae* has two growth requirements. The X factor, hemin, is a heat-stable substance associated with hemoglobin and directly available in sufficient quantity in routine sheep blood agar. The V factor (NAD) is a heat-labile coenzyme that can be supplied by adding yeast or potato extract to routine media. Alternately, certain bacteria such as staphylococci, neisseriae, pneumococci, and some other microorganisms synthesize the required NAD that enables *H. influenzae* satellitism. (Finegold et al.)

11. The specimen of choice for the isolation of *Bordetella pertussis* from a suspected case of whooping cough is

A. Blood
B. Cerebrospinal fluid
C. Nasopharyngeal swab
D. Throat swab

The answer is C. Whooping cough is an upper respiratory infection. Whereas a throat swab is sufficient for the recovery of some agents of upper respiratory infections, optimal recovery of *B. pertussis* is achieved by culture of a nasopharyngeal swab or aspirate. (Finegold et al.)

12. Family characteristics of the Enterobacteriaceae include

A. Fermentation of glucose
B. Fermentation of lactose
C. Production of indophenol oxidase
D. Failure to reduce nitrates

The answer is A. All species of the family Enterobacteriaceae are gram-negative rods that ferment glucose. Indophenol oxidase is not produced. Most species are capable of reducing nitrates to nitrites, but only some species ferment lactose. (Finegold et al.)

13. Twenty patients on a surgical ward develop urinary tract infections after catheterization. In each instance the isolated organism grows on sheep blood agar as a large, gray colony, and on MacConkey agar as a large, pink colony. The oxidase-negative gram-negative rod produces the same biotype and is resistant only to tetracycline. Additional biochemical results are as follows:

Phenylalanine deaminase (PAD): negative
Urease: negative
Hydrogen sulfide (H₂S): negative
Lysine decarboxylase: negative
Ornithine decarboxylase: positive
Indole: positive
Citrate: negative

The most probable identity of this organism is

A. *Escherichia coli*
B. *Enterobacter cloacae*
C. *Enterobacter aerogenes*
D. *Proteus vulgaris*

The answer is A. *E. coli*, the cause of this nosocomial outbreak, is one of the most frequent causes of hospital-acquired bacteriuria. Definitive identification of *E. coli* is confirmed by the PAD-negative, H₂S-negative, citrate-negative, indole-positive, urease-negative results. Both *Enterobacter* species are indole-negative and citrate-positive. *Proteus* species are PAD-positive and H₂S-positive. (Finegold et al.)

14. A mucoid, lactose-positive colony type on MacConkey agar that is indole-negative and citrate-positive is

A. *Escherichia coli*
B. *Klebsiella pneumoniae*
C. *Proteus vulgaris*
D. *Serratia marcescens*

The answer is B. *K. pneumoniae* is a lactose-positive, gram-negative rod on MacConkey agar. The IMViC reaction is $\theta\theta++$. Typical strains produce copious amounts of capsular polysaccharide that render the colony macroscopically mucoid. None of the alternative organisms are mucoid. *E. coli* has a positive indole and a negative citrate. *P. vulgaris* is lactose-negative on MacConkey agar, generally swarms on sheep blood agar, and has positive indole and citrate reactions. *S. marcescens* is lactose-negative on MacConkey agar (Lennette et al.)

15. *Escherichia*, *Klebsiella*, and *Proteus* species are frequently normal flora of the

A. Gastrointestinal tract
B. Respiratory tract

C. Superficial skin surfaces
D. Urinary tract

The answer is A. Many of the organisms of Enterobacteriaceae colonize the gastrointestinal tract, and as such, have been termed "coliforms." Among the commonly encountered Enterobacteriaceae, *Salmonella* and *Shigella* are notable in that they are never normal flora. The genera given in this question are all normal fecal flora. While they may be isolated from superficial skin surfaces, the respiratory or urinary tracts, they are not considered as normal microflora from these sites. (Finegold et al.)

16. A discharge from an infected ear grows a colorless colony type on MacConkey agar that swarms on sheep blood agar. This oxidase-negative, gram-negative rod is resistant to tetracycline and colistin on a routine Kirby-Bauer antimicrobial susceptibility test and gives the following biochemical reactions:

Phenylalanine deaminase (PAD): positive   Ornithine: positive
Hydrogen sulfide (H_2S): positive   Indole: negative
Urease: positive   Citrate: positive
Lysine: negative

The organism described is

A. *Citrobacter freundii*
B. *Morganella morganii*
C. *Proteus mirabilis*
D. *Proteus vulgaris*

The answer is C. Chronic otitis externa is usually associated with infection of pseudomonads or *Proteus* species. Here, the biochemical results confirm the presence of *P. mirabilis*. *C. freundii* is PAD-negative, *M. morganii* is H_2S-negative and indole-positive, and *P. vulgaris* is ornithine-negative and indole-positive. (Finegold et al.)

17. A gram-negative rod biochemically compatible with the genus *Salmonella* fails to agglutinate in the polyvalent somatic antisera for *Salmonella* serotyping. What is the next step in the definitive identification of this organism?

A. Report the organism as a *Salmonella* polyvalent O-positive species and send the isolate elsewhere for additional identification.
B. Wash a suspension of the isolate in saline and retest it in the *Salmonella* polyvalent antiserum.
C. Boil a saline suspension of the organism for 15 minutes, cool, and retype in *Salmonella* polyvalent antiserum.
D. Retest the isolate using the individual somatic antisera from each serogroup, A through E.

The answer is C. Occasional strains of *Salmonella* fail to agglutinate in polyvalent O antiserum. Some *Salmonella* species possess K antigens that render them nonagglutinable in the live, unheated form. These antigens can be inactivated by heating a saline suspension of the isolate at 100°C for at least 15 minutes. On retesting the cooled saline suspension in the *Salmonella* polyvalent antiserum, agglutination may occur. If agglutination occurs and group-specific antisera are available, individual grouping may be performed. Boiled suspensions that do not react in the polyvalent test may be *Salmonella* strains that belong to groups other than those represented in the typical polyvalent antiserum that includes groups A through E. (Lennette et al.)

18. A gram-negative rod is isolated from a patient with second- and third-degree burns. The isolate produces a bluish-green pigment and a characteristic "fruity" odor. Other characteristic observations are

Triple sugar iron: alk/alk   Oxidase: positive
Motility: positive   Oxidative/fermentation glucose:
                                  oxidative utilization only

The most probable genus of this isolate is

A. *Acinetobacter*
B. *Alcaligenes*
C. *Moraxella*
D. *Pseudomonas*

The answer is D. *Pseudomonas aeruginosa* is a probable infective agent in a burn patient. This organism is the only one that produces pyocyanin, a blue-green water-soluble pigment, and a fruity, grapelike odor. Although all pseudomonads are nonfermenters, most can utilize glucose oxidatively. Most pseudomonads produce indophenol oxidase, and are motile. *Alcaligenes* and *Moraxella* are nonsaccharolytic. *Acinetobacter* (*Herellea*) degrades glucose oxidatively but is oxidase-negative. *Acinetobacter* and *Moraxella* are nonmotile, and *Alcaligenes* is motile. (Finegold et al.)

19. After 48 hr of incubation on anaerobic sheep blood agar, *Clostridium perfringens* appears as a

A. Large, flat, fringy colony with a double zone of hemolysis
B. White, butyrous, nonhemolytic colony with a glistening surface
C. Gray, mucoid colony with a zone of alpha hemolysis
D. Colony with a pearl-like surface and a single zone of beta hemolysis

The answer is A. A double zone of hemolysis is typical for *C. perfringens*. The inner zone of complete hemolysis is distinct and surrounded by an indistinct zone of partial hemolysis. (Koneman et al.)

20. A *Bacteroides* species grows as a

A. Gram-negative rod on an anaerobic sheep blood agar plate
B. Gram-positive rod on an anaerobic sheep blood agar plate
C. Gram-negative rod on a capneic sheep blood agar plate
D. Gram-negative coccobacillus on a capneic sheep blood agar plate

The answer is A. Anaerobic sheep blood agar is used for the recovery of anaerobic bacteria. Therefore, an obligate anaerobic *Bacteroides* species will grow on the anaerobic sheep blood agar plate as a gram-negative rod. Sheep blood agar incubated in an increased CO_2 atmosphere is a nonselective, general-purpose plating medium for the isolation of facultative anaerobes. Capneic conditions do not support an anaerobe's growth. (Finegold et al.)

21. Isolation of *Campylobacter jejuni* from a patient with gastroenteritis is optimized by

A. Incubation at 35 to 37°C
B. Selective enrichment in selenite broth
C. A microaerophilic environment
D. An anaerobic environment without CO_2

The answer is C. *Campylobacter* species are oxidase-positive, curved gram-negative rods that can cause a wide spectrum of infections in humans. Gastrointestinal disease is associated with *C. jejuni*. This microbe is fastidious but grows on Skirrow's or supplemented Campy-blood agar medium. Broth enrichment of the specimen can be set up in Campy-thio. Selenite enrichment, which is recommended especially for the recovery of *Salmonella*, will not enhance the recovery of this microbe. Incubation at 42°C is desirable since *C. jejuni* thrives better at 42°C than at 35°C. Since this organism is a strict microaerophile, it grows best in an environment of less than 6% O_2. It also requires 5 to 10% CO_2. This atmosphere can be achieved easily by using the CampyPak microaerophilic generator envelope (BBL Microbiology Systems, Cockeysville, Md.) in a GasPak jar without a catalyst. Alternatively, evacuation and replacement of a jar with 5% O_2, 5% CO_2, and 90% N_2 gas mixture will achieve the desired environment. (Koneman et al.)

22. In the N-acetyl-L-cysteine–alkali method of processing sputum specimens for mycobacterial culture, the N-acetyl-L-cysteine serves as a

A. Buffer
B. Decontaminant
C. Digestant
D. pH stabilizer

The answer is C. N-acetyl-L-cysteine is a mucolytic agent that digests tenacious sputum specimens. Sodium hydroxide is a decontaminant. Phosphate buffer (pH 6.8) stabilizes the pH to stop the action of the N-acetyl-L-cysteine and sodium hydroxide solution. (Lennette et al.)

23. Acid-fast bacilli that grow at 35° C on Lowenstein-Jensen medium as rough, nonchromagenic mycobacteria that are niacin-positive and nitrate-positive are

   A. *Mycobacterium leprae*
   B. *Mycobacterium kansasii*
   C. *Mycobacterium scrofulaceum*
   D. *Mycobacterium tuberculosis*

The answer is D. *M. tuberculosis* is a slow-growing mycobacterium that typically produces a rough, buff-colored colony that is nonchromagenic in a light test for pigment production. Positive niacin and nitrate tests yield a definitive identification. (Lennette et al.)

24. Routine sterilization of artificial culture media by autoclaving is recommended at

   A. 15 psi at 121°C for 15 min
   B. 10 psi at 121°C for 10 min
   C. 15 psi at 200°F for 15 min
   D. 10 psi at 220°F for 10 min

The answer is A. Artificial culture media are routinely sterilized by moist heat under pressure of 15 psi at 121°C for 12 to 15 min. These conditions are sufficient to kill thermoresistant spore-forming bacilli commonly found in the laboratory environment. Overheating the medium can result in degradation of some of the basic nutrients in artificial media. Inadequate sterilization may result in contamination of the medium. (Finegold et al.)

25. When acetone-alcohol is inadvertently omitted from the Gram stain procedure, streptococci and neisseriae will be stained, respectively,

   A. Purple and red
   B. Purple and purple
   C. Red and red
   D. Red and purple

The answer is B. Iodine is a mordant that complexes with crystal violet and the cytoplasmic contents of bacteria. This complex cannot be eluted from gram-positive organisms such as streptococci because of their cell wall structure. Because of high lipid cell wall content in gram-negative organisms, acetone-alcohol treatment confers high permeability to the cell wall, which results in elution of the crystal violet complex. If the decolorizer is omitted, therefore, gram-negative bacteria such as neisseriae will remain purple. (Finegold et al.)

26. The color of a nonacid-fast bacillus following the acid-alcohol step and before counterstaining in the acid-fast stain procedure is

A. Blue
B. Red
C. Colorless
D. Green

The answer is C. Due to their high lipid content, acid-fast bacilli resist staining with ordinary dyes. Alcoholic basic aniline dyes are usually used to penetrate the cell. Depending on the method used, penetration may be augmented by the addition of heat or a wetting agent. After the initial staining step with carbolfuchsin, virtually all intact bacteria should appear red. Once stained, acid-fast bacilli resist decolorization with acid-alcohol and remain red. Most other bacteria are readily decolorized with acid-alcohol and appear colorless until a counterstain is applied. Methylene blue is commonly used to counterstain. (Finegold et al.)

27. MacConkey agar is used for the isolation of members of the family Enterobacteriaceae because the medium is

A. Inhibitory and differential
B. Differential and enriched
C. Enriched and selective
D. Selective and supplemented

The answer is A. MacConkey agar contains ingredients that select for Enterobacteriaceae and related gram-negative bacilli. That is, it contains bile salts and crystal violet, which inhibit the growth of gram-positive bacteria and some fastidious gram-negative bacilli. Additionally, this medium contains lactose and neutral red indicator, which make it differential for lactose fermentation, essential in the differentiation of enteric pathogens such as *Salmonella* and *Shigella*. (Koneman et al.)

28. Ethylhydrocupreine hydrochloride (optochin) is a chemical used to differentiate

A. Catalase-positive *Streptococcus* species from catalase-negative *Staphylococcus* species
B. *Streptococcus pneumoniae* from alpha-hemolytic streptococci
C. Enterobacteriaceae from non-Enterobacteriaceae
D. Group D enterococci from group D non-enterococci

The answer is B. Ethylhydrocupreine hydrochloride (optochin) is a quinine derivative that selectively inhibits the growth of *Str. pneumoniae*. Pneumococcal cells exposed to this chemical are lysed due to changes in surface tension, and a zone of inhibition greater than 14 mm results. Generally, the viridans streptococci are relatively resistant to optochin, resulting in no zone of inhibition. (Koneman et al.)

29. A lysine iron agar (LIA) slant shows a red slant over a yellow butt. This reaction indicates that the organism

 A. Deaminates lysine
 B. Decarboxylates lysine
 C. Ferments lactose
 D. Produces H$_2$S

The answer is A. LIA tests for fermentation of glucose, lysine decarboxylase (LDC), H$_2$S production, and lysine deaminase. Lysine deaminase is evidenced by a red slant reaction and indicates the tribe Proteeae. A yellow butt reveals fermentation of glucose with a negative LDC. Decarboxylation of lysine is evidenced by a purple butt reaction. H$_2$S formation results in the production of a black precipitate in the butt of the tube. (Finegold et al.)

30. Which of the following statements regarding Simmon's citrate agar is incorrect?

 A. Blue color is an alkaline reaction.
 B. Citrate is the only source of carbon in the medium.
 C. Glucose is the carbohydrate in the medium.
 D. Growth on the slant is interpreted as a positive reaction.

The answer is C. Simmon's citrate agar tests for the ability of an organism to utilize citrate as a sole source of carbon. Growth on the slant indicates this ability. Most organisms that grow will produce sufficient alkaline products to turn the bromthymol blue indicator from green to blue. Since the principle of this test is to determine the ability to utilize citrate as the only source of carbon, no other carbon-containing compounds, such as glucose, are ingredients in this medium. (Finegold et al.)

31. The reagent(s) used to detect a positive phenylalanine deaminase reaction is(are)

 A. Sulfanilic acid and alpha-naphthylamine
 B. p-Aminodimethylbenzaldehyde
 C. Alpha-naphthol and potassium hydroxide
 D. Ferric chloride

The answer is D. Phenylalanine deaminase deaminates the amino acid phenylalanine to phenylpyruvic acid. This alpha-keto acid forms a visible green-colored complex with 10% ferric chloride. Within the family Enterobacteriaceae only members of the tribe Proteeae possess the deaminase required to deaminate phenylalanine. (Koneman et al.)

32. To eliminate the antibacterial properties of blood and simultaneously introduce an adequate volume of blood for recovery of microorganisms from septicemia, the recommended blood-to-broth ratio in the blood culture bottle is approximately

A. 1:2
B. 2:1
C. 1:10
D. 10:1

The answer is C. A minimal blood dilution of 1:10 in blood culture broth virtually eliminates the inhibitory effect of previous antimicrobial chemotherapy on the recovery of microorganisms from the blood. Additionally, it dilutes the antibacterial properties of the serum. (Finegold et al.)

33. Which of the following specimens is acceptable for the evaluation of clinically important anaerobes?

A. Feces
B. Sputum
C. Synovial fluid
D. Superficial wound

The answer is C. Feces, sputa, and superficial wounds are frequently contaminated with normal microflora of the gastrointestinal tract, oropharyngeal area, and skin, respectively. Only those specimens that are likely to be devoid of contaminating organisms, such as synovial fluid, are acceptable for anaerobic evaluation. (Koneman et al.)

34. A urine is received in the laboratory for culture. If the specimen cannot be plated immediately, it should be held

A. In the freezer
B. In the refrigerator
C. At room temperature
D. In the 35°C incubator

The answer is B. Refrigeration is a practical and safe method to hold a urine specimen until it can be plated. In this manner, a urine may be held for up to 24 hr without significant alteration in bacterial population. It is paramount to refrigerate urine specimens immediately to avoid bacterial growth and significant increase in numbers of organisms in the urine. (Finegold et al.)

35. Standardized testing conditions for the Kirby-Bauer agar disk diffusion antimicrobial susceptibility test include all of the following *except*

A. Use of Mueller-Hinton media
B. Standard inoculum size
C. Incubation at 35°C
D. Incubation in 8 to 10% CO_2

The answer is D. Some testing variables that can affect the results of the Kirby-Bauer antimicrobial susceptibility test include composition of the medium, inoculum size, incubation conditions, and drug stability. Mueller-Hinton medium should be tested to assure that the medium pH is 7.2 to 7.4 and the approximate depth is 4 mm. Inoculum turbidity should be standardized to equal that of a No. 0.5 McFarland barium sulfate standard. Incubation of the plates at 35°C is recommended, since methicillin results are not reliable at 37°C. Because capneic incubation decreases the pH of the medium and affects the properties of some antimicrobials, aerobic incubation is required. (Lennette et al.)

36. The pair of organisms that would provide a good positive and negative control for phenylethyl alcohol (PEA) blood agar is

   A. *Pseudomonas aeruginosa* and *Escherichia coli*
   B. *Haemophilus influenzae* and *Streptococcus pyogenes*
   C. Enterococcus and *E. coli*
   D. *Staphylococcus aureus* and *Strept. pyogenes*

The answer is C. Phenylethyl alcohol agar is a selective medium for the isolation of gram-positive cocci including staphylococci and streptococci. This medium inhibits the growth of gram-negative bacteria. Since *E. coli* and *P. aeruginosa* are two gram-negative organisms, no positive growth control is included in option A. Similarly, no negative control is included in option D, since both organisms are gram-positive. Option B could be correct since it includes both a gram-negative and gram-positive organism; however, because the sheep blood enrichment of PEA does not support the growth of *H. influenzae*, it does not challenge the inhibitory characteristics of this medium. In option C an enterococcus species tests the PEA for ability to support growth and *E. coli* tests for the inhibition of growth. (*BBL Manual*)

37. Which of the following organisms will give the appropriate positive and negative reactions for quality control of the test listed?

	Positive	Negative
A. Gram stain	*Escherichia coli*	*Neisseria meningitidis*
B. Indole:	*E. coli*	*Proteus vulgaris*
C. Catalase	*Staphylococcus aureus*	*Staphylococcus epidermidis*
D. Oxidase	*Pseudomonas aeruginosa*	*E. coli*

The answer is D. Quality control requires that the performance of stains, media, and reagents be tested for the desired positive and negative reactions using stock culture strains of known stability. The performance characteristics of the oxidase reagent are tested adequately using *P. aeruginosa* as the positive control and *E. coli* as the negative control. Both *E. coli* and *N. meningitidis* are gram-negative. Both *E. coli* and *P. vulgaris* are indole-positive. Both *S. aureus* and *S. epidermidis* are catalase-positive. (Finegold et al.)

38. A fungal colony grows rapidly on Sabouraud's dextrose agar as a white colony type with a dense production of aerial, blue-green spores. On lactophenol cotton blue preparation, swollen-tipped conidiophores bear sterigmata and conidia in chains. The most likely identification of this isolate is

A. *Aspergillus*
B. *Helminthosporium*
C. *Penicillium*
D. *Scopulariopsis*

The answer is A. *Aspergillus* species are rapid-growing fungi that produce densely colored surfaces. Microscopically, septate, hyaline hyphae are seen, with swollen-tipped conidiophores. Sterigmata that radiate from the conidiophores bear chains of spherical conidia. *Penicillium* and *Scopulariopsis* produce freely branching, slender conidiophores of the "penicillus" type. *Helminthosporium* is a dematiaceous fungus. (Koneman et al.)

39. A saprobic yeast that inhabits airborne dust, skin, and mucosa grows rapidly and produces an orange-to-red color. This isolate most likely belongs to the genus

    A. *Cryptococcus*
    B. *Geotrichum*
    C. *Rhodotorula*
    D. *Saccharomyces*

The answer is C. *Rhodotorula* is a common yeast that is saprobic and found in airborne dust, skin, and mucosa. Cultures grow within 24 to 48 hr on Sabouraud's dextrose agar with colonies that are small, shiny, rounded, and orange-to-red. The color is due to carotenoid pigments that are produced by the genus. (Lennette et al.)

40. The function of 10% potassium hydroxide in the direct examination of skin, hair, and nail scrapings is to

    A. Preserve fungal elements
    B. Kill contaminating bacteria
    C. Clear and dissolve debris
    D. Fix preparation for subsequent staining

The answer is C. Direct examination of specimens submitted for fungal analysis can be crucial to early initiation of antifungal therapy. Ten % potassium hydroxide mounting fluid is recommended for the examination of skin, hair, and nail scrapings to clear and dissolve keratinous material that would render the preparation difficult to evaluate for fungal elements. (Koneman et al.)

41. A potentially pathogenic yeast that is normal flora in the oropharyngeal cavity and may produce thrush is

    A. *Aspergillus fumigatus*
    B. *Candida albicans*
    C. *Cryptococcus neoformans*
    D. *Rhizopus oryzae*

The answer is B. Although *Candida albicans* may be part of the normal oropharyngeal flora, oral candidiasis is commonly called thrush. *Cryptococcus neoformans* is another yeast that may rarely be part of the oropharyngeal flora, but it does not cause thrush. *A. fumigatus* and *R. oryzae* are true molds that are opportunistic pathogens of man. (Finegold et al.)

42. In an iodine preparation of feces, an amebic cyst appears to have a basket nucleus and a large glycogen mass that stains reddish-brown. The most probable identity of the cyst is

    A. *Entamoeba histolytica*
    B. *Iodamoeba bütschlii*
    C. *Naegleria fowleri*
    D. *Entamoeba hartmanni*

The answer is B. A cyst with the large, well-defined glycogen mass describes *I. bütschlii*. *Entamoeba* cysts have such masses only when very immature; however, these cysts have one to four nuclei and chromatoid bars, which are not present in *Iodamoeba* cysts. *N. fowleri* is found in tissues, not in stool contents. (Garcia et al.)

43. The infective stage of this parasite consists of an egg with a thin hyaline shell, with one flattened side and, usually, a fully developed larva within. The parasite is

    A. *Enterobius vermicularis*
    B. Hookworm
    C. *Ascaris lumbricoides*
    D. *Giardia lamblia*

The answer is A. *Enterobius* fits the description given in this item. Hookworm eggs are thin-shelled with an internal four- to eight-cell stage, which pulls away from the shell, resulting in an empty peripheral space. *Ascaris* has a thick shell with an albuminous coat that may be mamillated. *Giardia* cysts are oval with four nuclei within. (Koneman et al.)

44. The direct iodine preparation is best used to detect protozoan

    A. Eggs
    B. Trophozoites
    C. Cysts
    D. Larvae

The answer is C. Protozoan cysts stained with a weak iodine solution are refractile and show yellow-gold cytoplasm and brown glycogen. Although trophozoites also may be visible in iodine preparations, they are more easily detected by permanent stained slide or by their motility in unstained direct wet preparations. (Garcia et al.)

45. Parasites that are detected by direct visualization in a peripheral blood smear are

   A. *Ascaris*
   B. *Entamoeba*
   C. *Giardia*
   D. *Plasmodium*

The answer is D. *Plasmodium* species are the causative agents of malaria. Laboratory diagnosis of those bloodborne parasites involves preparing thick- and thin-film blood smears. Wright's or Giemsa stain may be used. *Ascaris*, *Entamoeba* and *Giardia* are generally intestinal tract parasites. (Finegold et al.)

46. Chlamydiae differ from viruses in that chlamydiae

   A. Are true bacteria
   B. Are obligate intracellular organisms
   C. Produce intracellular inclusions
   D. Are isolated in tissue culture systems

The answer is A. Chlamydiae have some characteristics in common with bacteria and some characteristics of viruses. Chlamydiae are bacteria that possess bacterialike cell walls and are gram-negative, although they usually cannot be visualized by Gram stain. Like viruses, chlamydiae are obligate intracellular organisms that can be visualized as intracellular inclusions using a Giemsa or Giménez stain. Similar to viruses, tissue culture techniques are required for growth and isolation. Unlike viruses that possess either RNA or DNA, chlamydiae contain both. (Lennette et al.)

47. A specimen for viral culture is collected on Friday and must be held for processing until Monday. In general, the optimal temperature for holding this specimen is

   A. 35°C
   B. 5°C
   C. −20°C
   D. −70°C

The answer is D. Specimens for viral isolation should be collected as soon as possible after the onset of the illness, preferably within 3 days, and refrigerated promptly. If processing will be performed within 24 hr, the specimen may be held at 4°C or on ice. To hold for long periods, the specimen should be frozen at −70°C. Freezing at −20°C is not recommended since some viruses are labile at this temperature. (Fenner and White)

48. A procedure that directly determines beta-lactamase production by a micro-organism is based on detection of a(n)

A. Zone of susceptibility around an ampicillin disk
B. Zone of inhibition around an oxacillin disk
C. Increased acidity due to the release of penicilloic acid
D. Increase in pH due to the reduction of iodine

The answer is C. The direct detection of beta-lactamase production is most commonly performed by demonstrating the ability of the microbe to convert penicillin to penicilloic acid. The rapid acidimetric method uses a pH indicator to detect the decrease in pH in response to cleavage of the beta-lactam ring to form penicilloic acid. The iodometric method centers on the ability of peni-cilloic acid to reduce iodine and, therein, decolorize a starch-iodine solution. Neither of the screening tests using ampicillin or oxacillin disks tests directly for beta-lactamase production. (Lennette et al.)

49. The antimicrobial testing protocol for gram-negative bacteria should rou-tinely include a disk impregnated with

A. Clindamycin
B. Erythromycin
C. Tobramycin
D. Oxacillin

The answer is C. Standard testing protocols for gram-negative bacteria rou-tinely include antimicrobials such as amikacin, ampicillin, carbenicillin, cephalosporins, gentamicin, tetracycline, tobramycin, and sulfamethoxazole-trimethroprim. Clindamycin, erythromycin, and vancomycin are used rou-tinely in gram-positive batteries. (Washington)

50. In a broth dilution method of antimicrobial susceptibility testing, the tube with the lowest concentration of antimicrobial in which there is no visible growth is the minimal

A. Antimicrobial concentration
B. Bacteriocidal concentration
C. Inhibitory concentration
D. Lethal concentration

The answer is C. The minimal inhibitory concentration (MIC) of an antimicro-bial is the lowest concentration of the drug that inhibits the growth of the organism as compared to a negative growth control. The minimal bacteriocidal concentration (MBC) is the lowest concentration of the drug that kills the organ-ism. The MBC is also known as the minimal lethal concentration (MLC). The minimal antimicrobial concentration has no meaning per se. (Finegold et al.)

CLS Review Questions

1. An early morning clean-catch midstream urine specimen yields these results on urinalysis:

Appearance: yellow, cloudy   Protein: 1+
Specific gravity: 1.025   Blood: negative
pH: 8.0   Ketones: negative
. Glucose: negative   Bilirubin: negative
Nitrite: positive
Microscopic: no casts, 15 to 25 WBCs per high-power field; many bacteria present

The results of this urinalysis indicate that

A. The bacteria present are the result of collection into a nonsterile container and correlate to a probable original count of less than 10^4 CFU per milliliter.
B. The bacteria present are the result of a delay of several hours in processing and correlate to probable original count of less than 10^4 CFU per milliliter.
C. Significant urinary tract infection that correlates to a probable original count of greater than 10^5 CFU per milliliter should be suspected.
D. Nephrotic syndrome should be considered, and the bacteria are merely coincidental.

The answer is C. The combination of a cloudy, concentrated (specific gravity ≥ 1.024), alkaline urine that is positive for nitrite and protein and in which WBCs are found on microscopic examination indicates probable urinary tract infection. Urine specimens that are not examined while fresh may deteriorate, and small numbers of contaminating bacteria can multiply, splitting urea, producing nitrite, and increasing the pH. However, large numbers of WBCs would not be found in that instance. Large numbers of WBCs without an alkaline pH and positive nitrite reaction may indicate either an inflammation without infection or a short urine transit time during which significant bacterial growth has not occurred. (Ross et al.)

2. This adult disease is more appropriately considered an intoxication than an infection because the preformed neurotoxin that is ingested causes the symptoms of neuromuscular paralysis. The agent that produces the toxin is

A. *Bacillus cereus*
B. *Clostridium botulinum*
C. *Clostridium tetani*
D. *Staphylococcus aureus*

The answer is B. The spores of *C. botulinum* occur in the soil ubiquitously. Intoxication in adults results from consumption of inadequately preserved foods in which spores of *C. botulinum* germinate and produce the neurotoxin.

In this country, the incriminated foods are usually canned vegetables. Infant botulism is a special case resulting from ingestion of the spores with subsequent colonization of the intestinal tract and production of the toxin in situ. *S. aureus* food poisoning results from ingestion of preformed enterotoxin and causes severe vomiting and diarrhea. Ingestion of *B. cereus*–contaminated food results in a profuse, watery diarrhea. *C. tetani* causes tetanus (lockjaw), which manifests with classical neuromuscular symptoms. However, the pathogenesis requires a deep tissue wound, contaminated with soil-containing spores, that becomes necrotic and sufficiently deoxygenated to allow proliferation of the organism. Once the primary *C. tetani* infection is established, the neurotoxin tetanospasmin is produced and spreads to the central nervous system where neuromuscular symptoms result. (Lennette et al.)

3. Two siblings arrive at the emergency room. Both had antecedent sore throats about 2 to 3 weeks earlier that grew beta-hemolytic streptococci; now they present with different clinical symptoms. The brother displays edema and hypertension, and RBC casts are seen in the urine. The sister complains of fever and joint pains and has carditis. The diseases that these siblings have are most likely

    A. Erysipelas and glomerulonephritis
    B. Glomerulonephritis and rheumatic fever
    C. Rheumatic fever and scarlet fever
    D. Scarlet fever and erysipelas

The answer is B. Although beta-hemolytic streptococcus, group A can cause several types of disease, it most commonly causes an infection of the pharynx and adjacent areas. Symptoms from *Streptococcus pyogenes* arise initially from an acute upper respiratory infection. If inadequately treated, delayed complications can result, such as the two cardinal sequelae described in these siblings. The sister exhibits rheumatic fever, in which carditis and arthritic joints are major features. The brother displays acute glomerulonephritis with typical kidney pathology. Erysipelas and scarlet fever are skin manifestations of *S. pyogenes*. Erysipelas is an inflammatory skin disease in which large numbers of streptococci are present in the periphery of the lesions. Scarlet fever is a superificial skin rash resulting from the production of the unique scarlatinal toxin. (Volk)

4. Purulent material is obtained from a carbuncle and submitted for bacterial culture. The direct smear reveals many gram-positive cocci and WBCs. The culture shows growth in the primary broth and on the sheep blood agar plate and no growth on the MacConkey agar plate. The colonies on the blood agar plate are butyrous, white, and beta-hemolytic. Both glucose and mannitol are fermented. Although the slide coagulase test is negative, the tube coagulase test is positive. The most probable identity of this isolate is

    A. *Micrococcus lysodeikticus*
    B. *Staphylococcus aureus*

C. *Staphylococcus epidermidis*
D. *Staphylococcus saprophyticus*

The answer is B. *S. aureus* is a gram-positive coccus frequently isolated from this site. The positive coagulase tube test, which demonstrates the presence of "free" coagulase, is the best test to identify *S. aureus* definitively. Not all strains of *S. aureus* possess "bound" coagulase, as evidenced in the data by the negative slide coagulase test. Most strains of *S. aureus* also ferment mannitol. Micrococci do not utilize glucose anaerobically. Staphylococci other than *S. aureus* are coagulase-negative. (Finegold et al.)

7. A gram-negative coccobacillary organism that is isolated from synovial fluid on chocolate agar resembles either a *Moraxella* species or *Neisseria gonorrhoeae*. The single best test to distinguish between these organisms is

   A. Beta hemolysis
   B. Glucose degradation
   C. Motility
   D. Oxidase production

The answer is B. *Moraxella* species and *N. gonorrhoeae* can be isolated from similar specimen sources such as the genitourinary tract, blood, and synovial fluid. The micromorphology of *Moraxella* is coccobacillary, sometimes resembling a gonococcus. The single best test for distinguishing *N. gonorrhoeae* from a *Moraxella* species is carbohydrate degradation. *N. gonorrhoeae* forms acid from glucose, whereas *Moraxella* species are metabolically inactive in carbohydrate utilization tests. Both *Neisseria* and *Moraxella* produce indophenol oxidase and are nonmotile. *Moraxella* species are nonhemolytic on sheep blood agar. Because *N. gonorrhoeae* does not routinely grow on sheep blood agar, beta hemolysis is irrelevant. (Lennette et al.)

8. A lumbar puncture is performed on an 82-year-old woman who is receiving immunosuppressive therapy. The direct Gram stain of the CSF reveals small gram-positive rods and numerous WBCs. At 18 hr, a small translucent colony type grows on sheep blood agar with a narrow zone of beta hemolysis. Identification of this isolate could be made by demonstration of

   A. Tumbling motility
   B. Metachromatic granulation
   C. Hippurate hydrolysis
   D. Capsule formation

The answer is A. *Listeria monocytogenes* is a small gram-positive rod often associated with meningitis in infants and elderly adults. The organism is an opportunistic pathogen in patients with predisposing conditions such as malignancies and blood dyscrasias, and, as in this instance, in patients receiving immunosuppressive therapy. Growth on sheep blood agar yields small, round translucent colonies with a faintly detectable narrow zone of beta hemolysis. Key characteristics for the identification of *L. monocytogenes* include blackening of routine bile esculin agar, tumbling motility at 25°C, and development of an umbrella-like area of motility in a semisolid medium incubated at 25°C. Metachromatic granulation is a characteristic attribute of *Corynebacterium diphtheriae*. The ability to hydrolyze hippurate is a characteristic of *Streptococcus agalactiae*. The ability to form a capsule is not an attribute of *L. monocytogenes*. (Finegold et al.)

9. An acute infectious respiratory outbreak occurs in the overcrowded poverty-stricken central core of a United States–Mexico border town. A 5-year-old girl was admitted to the city hospital 48 hr ago and has expired. Her 7-year-old brother was admitted as a prime candidate in the epidemic. Physical examination of this child reveals fever and pseudomembranous, white patchy spots in the pharynx, but no sore throat. The probable diagnosis is

   A. Diphtheria
   B. Epiglottitis
   C. Pertussis
   D. Trench mouth

The answer is A. The infectious outbreak described is consistent with diphtheria. Diphtheria is an acute infection in which the organisms localize in the oropharyngeal area multiplying in number to produce the notorious pseudomembrane and exotoxin. It is the diphtherial exotoxin that causes myocarditis and congestive heart failure. At risk are unimmunized children who in this country are likely to inhabit crowded border towns or central-city ghettos. Treatment for active cases involves the administration of specific antitoxin as soon as possible. (Lennette et al.)

10. A dairy farmer who has an intermittent fever, progressive weakness, and night sweats is suspected of having undulant fever. A likely etiologic agent that requires an atmosphere of 10% CO_2 and is urease-positive in 1 to 2 hr is

    A. *Bacillus anthracis*
    B. *Bacillus cereus*
    C. *Brucella abortus*
    D. *Brucella melitensis*

The answer is C. Brucellosis in cattle causes contagious abortion, or Bang's disease, and commonly results from infection with *Brucella abortus*. Undulant fever in humans is a generalized infection with several typical clinical manifestations, one of which is described above.

   B. abortus is the only *Brucella* species that requires up to 10% CO_2 for primary isolation. It also is urease-positive in 1 to 2 hr. *Brucella melitensis* is most often found in sheep and goats, does not require CO_2 for growth, and varies in its ability to split urea. *Bacillus anthracis* is the etiologic agent of anthrax in cattle and, secondarily, in humans. *Bacillus cereus* causes food poisoning in humans. (Lennette et al.)

11. A patient is admitted to the hospital with symptoms of appendicitis. A stool specimen for culture reveals a gram-negative bacillus that is oxidase-negative, catalase-positive, urease-positive, and weakly fermentative. The slant of Kligler's iron agar (KIA) is orange-yellow. These reactions suggest the possibility of

A. *Yersinia enterocolitica*
B. *Escherichia coli*
C. *Plesiomonas shigelloides*
D. *Pasteurella multocida*

The answer is A. *Y. enterocolitica* and *Yersinia pseudotuberculosis* are capable of causing a mesenteric lymphadenitis that clinically simulates appendicitis. The genus *Yersinia* differs from the genera *Pasteurella* and *Plesiomonas* in that *Yersinia* is cytochrome oxidase–negative whereas *Pasteurella* and *Plesiomonas* are oxidase-positive. The positive urease reaction differentiates *Yersinia* from *E. coli*. Sucrose fermentation distinguishes the two species of *Yersinia*. *Y. enterocolitica* ferments sucrose and *Y. pseudotuberculosis* does not. (Finegold, et al.)

12. A stool culture from an adult appears to have two lactose-negative colony types on Hektoen and xylose-lysine-deoxycholate agar. One colony type retains the original color of each medium and the other has black centers. Stool screen data are as follows:

Medium	Isolate 1	Isolate 2
Triple sugar iron (TSI)	Alkaline/acid, no gas, H_2S-negative	Acid/acid, gas, H_2S-positive
Lysine iron agar (LIA)	Lysine-negative, H_2S-negative	Red slant, lysine-negative, H_2S-positive
Urease	Negative	Positive

Based on these data and additional biochemical testing, an important step is to

A. Set up enteropathogenic *Escherichia coli* agglutinations.
B. Set up *Shigella* agglutinations.
C. Set up *Salmonella* agglutinations.
D. Report the culture as negative for enteropathogens.

The answer is B. The stool screen reactions for isolate 1 are typical of those expected for a *Shigella* species. However, they are also consistent with a possible lysine-negative *E. coli* or *Aeromonas hydrophila*; therefore, biochemical confirmation and *Shigella* agglutination should be performed for this isolate. Agglutinations for enteropathogenic *E. coli* are unnecessary for adults. Since the stool screen on isolate 2 indicates reactions that are typical for a *Proteus* species, no additional workup is necessary for this isolate. (Finegold et al.)

13. Both blood and urine cultures are positive for an oxidase-negative, gram-negative rod that is colorless on MacConkey's agar. Biochemical reactions include the following:

Phenylalanine deaminase: negative   DNase: positive
H₂S: negative   Arabinose: alkaline
Indole: negative   Lysine decarboxylase: positive
Citrate: positive   Ornithine decarboxylase: positive
Rhamnose: alkaline

This organism, an opportunistic pathogen, should be susceptible to

A. Ampicillin
B. Cephalothin
C. Polymyxin B
D. Gentamicin

The answer is D. This patient's blood and urine cultures are positive for the opportunist *Serratia marcescens*. The biochemical reactions are all typical and the positive DNase or alkaline rhamnose, coupled with the alkaline arabinose reaction, pinpoints the identification. The typical antibiogram for *Serratia marcescens* shows resistance to ampicillin, cephalothin, and polymyxin B. Gentamicin is the drug of choice for this organism. (Finegold, et al., Lennette et al.)

14. The metabolism of glucose by the *Klebsiella-Enterobacter-Serratia* group is as follows:

$$\text{Glucose} \rightarrow 2,3\text{-butanediol} + 2\ CO_2 + H_2$$

The reaction is the basis for the

A. Glucose oxidase reaction
B. Methyl red test
C. Oxidative/fermentation (O-F) glucose test
D. Voges-Proskauer test

The answer is D. All members of the family Enterobacteriaceae metabolize glucose to pyruvate via the Embden-Meyerhof pathway. The subsequent metabolism of pyruvate results in either mixed organic acid end products or the formation of neutral 2,3-butanediol end product. In the methyl red test mixed acid end products decrease the acidity of the medium to approximately pH 4.4, where the methyl red indicator in the medium is red. In the Voges-Proskauer test, the neutral 2,3-butanediol end product is detected by a colorimetric reaction. The Klebsielleae utilize the butylene-glycol pathway, which results in a negative methyl red test and a positive Voges-Proskauer test. (Koneman et al.)

15. A stool specimen is submitted for culture from a patient with gastro-enteritis, nausea, and vomiting. A gram-negative rod grows on thiosulfate

citrate bile salts sucrose agar (TCBS) as a large green colony type. Additional screening characteristics include

Triple sugar iron (TSI): alk/acid   Catalase: positive
H_2S: negative   Nitrate: positive
Oxidase: positive   Lysine: positive

The most probable presumptive identification of this isolate is

A. *Aeromonas hydrophila*
B. *Shigella flexneri*
C. *Vibrio parahaemolyticus*
D. *Yersinia enterocolitica*

The answer is C. TCBS is an excellent selective and differential medium for the isolation of vibrios. Most fecal flora and gastrointestinal pathogens are inhibited on this medium. *V. parahaemolyticus* appears as a large, blue-green colony on TCBS agar at 24 hr of incubation. Key characteristics include TSI-alk/acid, oxidase-positive, and lysine-positive reactions. *Shigella* and *Yersinia* are oxidase-negative and lysine-negative. Although *Aeromonas* is oxidase-positive, it is lysine-negative. (Koneman et al.; Finegold et al.)

16. A patient specimen from an endotrachael intubation reveals a nonmotile gram-negative coccobacillary rod that grows on MacConkey agar as a lactose-negative colony at 24 hr. It is a nonfermentative organism. A large battery of conventional biochemicals yields the following reactions:

OF: glucose (aerobic): acid   Lactose: alkaline
OF: glucose (anaerobic):   Maltose: alkaline
   alkaline   Mannitol: alkaline
Oxidase: negative   Sucrose: alkaline
TSI: alkaline/no change   Xylose: acid
Orthonitrophenyl galactoside (ONPG): negative

This isolate also produces acid from a 10% lactose agar slant. The identification of this isolate is

A. *Acinetobacter (Herellea)*
B. *Alcaligenes faecalis*
C. *Moraxella osloensis*
D. *Pseudomonas cepacia*

The answer is A. This isolate is *Acinetobacter calcoaceticus* var. *anitratus*, with the common name, *Herellea*. *Herellea* is a nonmotile coccobacillary gram-negative nonfermentative microbe. Its key reactions using the King criteria are glucose oxidizer, MacConkey-positive, and oxidase-negative. Typical reactions include the production of acid from OF xylose and a 10% lactose slant. *Alcaligenes faecalis* is nonsaccharolytic and motile with peritrichous flagellation. *M. osloensis* is nonsaccharolytic and nonmotile. Although *P. cepacia* is an oxidizer, it is motile with polar flagellation, and it is ONPG-positive. (Lennette et al.)

17. Which result is *not* consistent with the identification of *Mycobacterium fortuitum?*

    A. Arylsulfatase positive
    B. Niacin positive
    C. Growth on MacConkey agar
    D. Growth in 5% NaCl

The answer is B. *M. fortuitum* may be differentiated from the other rapid-growing mycobacteria by its positive arylsulfatase reaction within 3 to 5 days and its growth on MacConkey agar within 5 days. This saprobe also grows in 5% NaCl in 3 to 5 days. Although niacin may aid in distinguishing between *M. fortuitum* and *Mycobacterium chelonei*, niacin accumulation varies among strains of *M. chelonei*. (Finegold et al.)

18. An acid-fast bacillus (AFB) has been isolated from the sputum of a patient suspected to have a mycobacterial pulmonary disease. The organism is a slow-growing isolate that produces cream- to tan-colored colonies when grown in the dark in the incubator and after exposure to light. This organism is most likely which of the following mycobacteria?

    A. *Mycobacterium avium-intracellulare* complex
    B. *Mycobacterium chelonei*
    C. *Mycobacterium kansasii*
    D. *Mycobacterium scrofulaceum*

The answer is A. Mycobacteria that are slow-growing nonphotochromogens include the TB complex, *M. ulcerans*, and the Runyon group III species. The *M. avium-intracellulare* complex includes AFB in Runyon group III, capable of causing serious pulmonary disease similar to tuberculosis. *M. chelonei* is a Runyon group IV rapid grower. *M. kansasii* and *M. scrofulaceum* are slow-growing AFB that are group I photochromogens and group II scotochromogens, respectively. (Finegold et al.)

19. *Nocardia* species that cause nocardiosis often are

    A. Obligate anaerobes
    B. Gram-variable
    C. Partially acid-fast
    D. Spore-forming rods

The answer is C. *Nocardia* species are nonspore-forming, branching, gram-positive bacilli. They are characterized as being partially acid-fast; i.e., they retain the carbolfuchsin when decolorized with a diluted acid-alcohol solution. *Nocardia* species are generally aerobic, although they tend toward micro-aerophilic or capnophilic requirements. (Finegold et al.)

20. A direct Gram stain of a pelvic mass from a patient with an IUD shows numerous pus cells and branching, beaded, gram-positive rods. Heaped, lobate colonies grow anaerobically and develop a "molar-tooth" appearance after several days of incubation. The most probable identity is

A. *Actinomyces israelii*
B. *Mycobacterium phlei*
C. *Nocardia asteroides*
D. *Trichosporon capitatum*

The answer is A. The description of the anaerobic, branched, gram-positive rods is typical of *Actinomyces*. *A. israelii* develops mature molar-tooth-type colonies, has been shown to be present in the cervix of approximately 5 to 25% of women using IUDs, and has been implicated in pelvic infections complicated by IUDs. None of the other three alternatives are anaerobes. (Finegold et al.)

21. A lung abscess is cultured. At 24 hr of capneic incubation, no growth is detected on any of the primary agar plates. Gram-negative rods are seen in the thioglycollate broth. After 48 hr, the growth includes

Anaerobic sheep blood agar: 3+ gram-negative rods
Anaerobic laked blood agar with kanamycin-vancomycin (K-V): 3+ gram-negative rods

The isolate fluoresces a brick-red color under long-wave ultraviolet exposure. If allowed to incubate several more days, the colonies would be visibly

A. Black-pigmented
B. Yellow-pigmented
C. Orange-pigmented
D. Blue-pigmented

The answer is A. Anaerobic gram-negative rods that are initially nonpigmented on laked blood agar with K-V and fluoresce brick-red when exposed to ultraviolet light (365 nm) are of the *Bacteroides melaninogenicus* group. With age, the fluorescence disappears and a brown-black pigment is produced. These bacteria are important pathogens in respiratory infections and are seen in other infections as well. (Washington)

22. Two organisms that are thought to act synergistically to produce an ulcerative infection of the gums, commonly called trench mouth, are

A. *Treponema pertenue* and *Streptococcus mitis*
B. *Streptococcus mitis* and *Fusobacterium nucleatum*
C. *Fusobacterium necrophorum* and *Borrelia vincentii*
D. *Borrelia vincentii* and *Treponema pertenue*

The answer is C. This ulcerative or pseudomembranous infection of the gums is thought to be a "fusospirochetal disease" related to *B. vincentii* and *F.*

necrophorum. Demonstration of Vincent's infection can be made by staining smears with Gram's crystal violet for 1 min and examining them for the presence of numerous white cells and fusospirochetal organisms. Culture of mouth lesions or pseudomembrane is of no value. (Finegold et al.)

23. A physician inquires about repeated sputum specimens, negative on routine bacterial culture, that are reported to contain only normal oropharyngeal flora. The patient is a 67-year-old man who smokes 15 to 20 cigarettes a day and has persistent cough, malaise, and a fever of 102 to 105°F. Treatment with routine antimicrobials such as penicillin and cephalothin has not been effective; the cough and fever persist. The most recent direct Gram stain of sputum shows 3+ PMNs, mucus present, and rare epithelial cells. A likely etiologic agent is

   A. *Haemophilis influenzae*
   B. *Legionella pneumophila*
   C. *Pseudomonas aeruginosa*
   D. *Streptococcus pneumoniae*

The answer is B. Repeatedly negative sputum cultures from an elderly patient who smokes, has pneumonia with persistent cough and high fever, and does not respond to routine drug therapy are suggestive of legionellosis. Definitive diagnosis requires isolation of the organism from the lung tissue on a special medium, such as buffered charcoal yeast extract agar, or a rapid immunodiagnostic approach. Erythromycin is the drug of choice. *H. influenzae* is seldom the causative agent of adult pneumonia and should grow on chocolate agar on routine sputum culture. Both *P. aeruginosa* and *S. pneumoniae* can be recovered from routine sputum cultures. (Volk; Finegold et al.)

24. Which of the following descriptions characterize *Pasteurella multocida?*

   A. Gram-negative coccoid bacillus
   B. Growth on MacConkey agar
   C. Beta-hemolytic on sheep blood agar
   D. Obligate anaerobe

The answer is A. *P. multocida* is a small coccobacillary gram-negative rod that is a facultative anaerobe. It grows on sheep blood agar as a small translucent colony type that is nonhemolytic and fails to grow on MacConkey agar. Among the pasteurellae, *P. haemolytica* is beta-hemolytic on blood agar and grows on MacConkey agar, and *P. aerogenes* grows on MacConkey agar. (Finegold et al.)

25. Which of the following media has a high protein content and requires sterilization by inspissation?

   A. Löwenstein-Jensen egg
   B. Sheep blood agar
   C. Thioglycollate
   D. Christensen's urease

The answer is A. Inspissation is a moist heat method of sterilization in which the medium thickens by coagulation and evaporation when exposed to a temperature of 75°C on 3 consecutive days for 2 hr each day. This sterilization method is generally used to avoid altering the appearance of media that contain high amounts of protein, egg, or serum. Thioglycollate is autoclaved routinely; sterile sheep blood is added to basal agar after autoclaving; and urea must be filter-sterilized for incorporation into Christensen's urease. (Finegold et al.)

26. All of the following describe the orthonitrophenyl galactoside (ONPG) test *EXCEPT*

    A. It detects the presence or absence of the enzyme beta-galactosidase in an organism.
    B. It is positive for organisms that are pink or red on MacConkey agar, and negative for those that are colorless on MacConkey agar at 24 hr.
    C. It is positive for isolates that are capable of fermenting lactose, but lack the permease.
    D. It detects the decarboxylation of ONPG to ornithine and galactose.

The answer is D. Rapid lactose-fermenting bacteria possess two enzymes: lactose permease enhances transport of lactose across the cell wall, and beta-galactosidase cleaves the galactoside bond of lactose, producing glucose and galactose. The glucose is then degraded by the Embden-Meyerhof pathway, producing mixed acid fermentation. In conventional lactose fermentation tests, such as that using MacConkey agar, both enzymes must be present to evidence a rapid positive test. Some species appear to be nonlactose fermenters at 18 to 24 hr because they lack the permease activity, even though they possess beta-galactosidase. Because ONPG readily permeates the cell and is structurally similar to lactose, the ONPG test detects only beta-galactosidase activity. By circumventing the need for permease, ONPG rapidly identifies these late lactose-fermenting bacteria. (Koneman et al.)

27. Bacteria that are glucose oxidizers in Hugh-Leifson (H-L) OF medium produce an alkaline/no change reaction in Kligler iron agar (KIA) because

    A. These organisms produce insufficient amounts of acid to be detected on KIA.
    B. The lactose component in KIA inhibits glucose oxidation in this medium.
    C. The concentration of glucose in KIA is higher than in the OF medium.
    D. KIA detects only fermentation of lactose.

The answer is A. Fermentation media such as KIA contain 2% peptone and 0.1% glucose. In contrast, Hugh-Leifson OF medium contains 0.2% peptone and 1% glucose or other carbohydrate. The decrease in peptone reduces the formation of alkaline end products from oxidation of amino acids. The increase in carbohydrate enhances production of acids. Consequently, H-L OF medium is a more sensitive medium for detecting weak acid production.

Nonfermentative bacteria, such as *Pseudomonas aeruginosa*, which utilize glucose oxidatively, produce small amounts of acid in H-L OF medium exposed to air. Because KIA contains a low concentration of glucose, these organisms resort to oxidative utilization of peptone to form amines that result in an alkaline/no change reaction on KIA. (Finegold et al.)

28. Physical examination of a 20-year-old man seen in the emergency room reveals nuchal rigidity and a temperature of 102°F. Direct Gram stain of the CSF reveals numerous WBCs and a few gram-negative diplococci. The isolate grows on sheep blood agar and is oxidase-positive. Acid production occurs in the cystine trypticase agar (CTA) carbohydrates as follows:

Glucose: acid
Lactose: acid
Maltose: acid
Sucrose: acid

The most appropriate action to take is

A. Identify the organism as meningococcus and report it.
B. Identify the organism as *Moraxella* and set up additional tests to determine the species.
C. Gram-stain and subculture the CTA sugars to check them for purity.
D. Perform an antimicrobial susceptibility test as a confirmation of the identification.

The answer is C. This situation represents a classic presentation of meningococcal meningitis, diagnosed on the basis of clinical symptoms and preliminary culture results. Because meningococci ferment glucose and maltose exclusively, and *Moraxella* species are unable to attack carbohydrates, it appears that the CTA sugars are contaminated. The possibility that the sugars contain more than the patient's isolate could be established by Gram stain and subculture. Antimicrobial susceptibility testing does not aid identification when the carbohydrate reactions are discrepant. (Koneman et al.)

29. Blood cultures should be incubated more than 7 days if the differential diagnosis includes all of the following *except*

A. Brucellosis
B. Candidemia
C. Gonococcemia
D. Typhoid fever

The answer is D. Blood cultures should be held for more than 7 days for any of the first three diagnoses. Blood is the best specimen for recovery of *Brucella* during the febrile illness. Castañeda bottles with CO_2 are recommended for incubation; the culture should be incubated at least 21 days and subcultured periodically before reported as negative. With candidemia and fungemia the organisms often do not grow rapidly in routine blood culture media and may require up to 2 weeks incubation. Similarly, in gonococcemia small numbers of sequestered organisms and slow growth rates render it advisable to hold blood culture bottles 7 to 14 days. However, most bacteria are present in numbers large enough and grow rapidly such that detection of growth is possible within the first few days of incubation. (Finegold et al.)

30. Safety precautions designed to minimize laboratory-acquired infections when working with *Mycobacterium tuberculosis* in a clinical laboratory would prevent spreading of these organisms by

    A. Aerosol production
    B. Ingestion
    C. Superficial contact
    D. Contact with fomites

The answer is A. Tuberculosis is initiated by inhalation of droplet nuclei of less than 5 μm. Inhalation of infectious aerosols is the major biohazard to microbiology laboratory personnel. To minimize laboratory-acquired infection, safety precautions are designed that prevent spread of aerosols and inhalation of droplet nuclei. (Lennette et al.)

31. To check for positive and negative reactions, select the appropriate set of quality control microorganisms for the following tests:

    Bile esculin hydrolysis   6.5% NaCl tolerance
    Bacitracin susceptibility   Hippurate hydrolysis

    A. *Streptococcus pyogenes*, viridans streptococcus, enterococcus
    B. *Str. pyogenes*, *Streptococcus agalactiae*, enterococcus
    C. *Staphylococcus aureus*, *Str. pyogenes*, enterococcus
    D. *Str. agalactiae*, viridans streptococcus, enterococcus

The answer is B. An appropriate quality control set of microorganisms would be as follows:

Test	Positive Reaction	Negative Reaction
Bile esculin hydrolysis	Enterococcus	*Str. pyogenes*
Bacitracin susceptibility	*Str. pyogenes*	*Str. agalactiae*
6.5% NaCl tolerance	Enterococcus	*Str. pyogenes*
Hippurate hydrolysis	*Str. agalactiae*	*Str. pyogenes*
(Henry)		

32. From the dimorphic fungi and major identifying morphologic features listed, select the species whose major characteristics are *not* described correctly.

    A. *Blastomyces dermatitidis*: thick-walled yeast cells with single, broad-based buds at 37°C
    B. *Coccidioides immitis*: barrel-shaped arthrospores at 25°C
    C. *Histoplasma capsulatum*: spherical, tuberculated macroaleuriospores at 25°C
    D. *Sporothrix schenckii*: thick-walled yeast cells with multiple buds at 25°C

The answer is D. The morphologic features of the dimorphic molds that cause disease in humans are of major importance in determining the etiology of these sometimes life-threatening illnesses. Pertinent criteria of the thermally dimorphic species are as follows:

Blastomyces dermatitidis: at 37°C tan- to cream-colored colonies with wrinkled surfaces and waxy sheen; microscopically, large, thick-walled yeast cells that have single buds attached by a broad base

Coccidioides immitis: at room temperature, white-to-brown colonies with cottony aerial mycelia; microscopically, septate hyphae dissociate and fragment into barrel-shaped arthrospores

Histoplasma capsulatum: at room temperature, silky-smooth, white-to-tan colonies; microscopically, echinate, tuberculated, spherical macroaleuriospores (macroconidia)

Sporothrix schenckii: at room temperature, smooth cream-to-white colonies that turn brown with age; microscopically, branched slender conidiophores with small conidia arranged in "flowerettes" and/or in a "sleeve" arrangement

(Koneman et al.)

33. *Fusarium* species have on occasion been associated with corneal ulcers, ulcerated skin conditions, and mycetoma. Typical macromorphologic and micromorphologic features are:

   A. Rapid growers that usually produce a lavender pigment and crescent-shaped, septate macroconidia
   B. Rapid growers that darken with age and produce aseptate hyphae with rhizoids
   C. Slow growers that are velvety and light tan, with a salmon-colored reverse, and seldom produce macroconidia
   D. Slow growers that are gray-brown and produce multicellular macroconidia with both transverse and longitudinal septa

The answer is A. *Fusarium* is a genus of fungi that is pathogenic to plants. Commonly considered a contaminant, it is known to cause keratomycosis and mycetoma. Its colonies are cottony on Sabouraud's dextrose agar, with a lavender pigment at 4 days. Microscopically, it is a septate hyaline fungus that produces crescent-shaped septate macroconidia. Option B describes the member of Zygomycetes, *Rhizopus*. Option C describes the dermatophyte *Microsporum audouinii*. Option D describes the dematiaceous fungus *Alternaria*. (Finegold et al.; Lennette et al.)

34. An 8-year-old child presents with tinea capitis, thought to be caused by *Microsporum canis*. Suspicions can be confirmed by

   A. Direct examination of infected hair for fluorescence under a Wood's lamp
   B. Demonstration of endothrix invasion of hair
   C. Salmon-colored reverse of colony
   D. Production of abundant microaleuriospores on Sabouraud's dextrose agar

The answer is A. *M. canis* is a common agent of ringworm in domestic animals and of tinea capitis in children in the United States. Most human infections are acquired from cats and dogs. Hairs infected with a species of *Microsporum* fluoresce a bright yellow-green under ultraviolet examination. Most other dermatophytes do not fluoresce. Many dermatophytes have a predilection for ectothrix—infection of hair evidenced by conidia forming a sheath around the surface of the hair shaft. *Microsporum* grows on Sabouraud's dextrose agar as a white, fluffy colony type with a chrome-yellow reverse. Microscopic examination of the colony reveals thick-walled, echinate, spindle-shaped macroaleuriospores, usually with an asymmetric terminal knob. *M. canis* can be differentiated from *Microsporum audouinii* by the ability of *M. canis* to grow and sporulate on polished rice grains. (Finegold et al.; Lennette et al.)

35. Which of the following pairings of yeast species with identifying characteristics is (are) correct?

   A. *Cryptococcus neoformans*: urease-negative, encapsulated
   B. *Candida albicans*: germ tube–negative, chlamydospore producer
   C. *Torulopsis glabrata*: urease-positive, arthroconidia producer
   D. *Geotrichum* species: hyphae-positive, arthroconidia producer

The answer is D. There are several approaches to laboratory identification of yeasts. Some key characteristics and preliminary tests are as follows:

Germ tube test: positive for *Candida albicans* in 2 hr and negative for most of the yeast species in this time limit
Urease test: positive for *Cryptococcus* and *Rhodotorula* and negative for *Torulopsis, Geotrichum,* and *Candida* species, except for an occasional strain of *Candida krusei*
India ink test: positive for encapsulated yeast such as *Cryptococcus neoformans* and negative for nonencapsulated yeast species
Corn meal agar: detects formation of chlamydospores, arthroconidias, and blastoconidia; *Candida albicans* forms chlamydospores, *Geotrichum* forms hyphae and arthroconidia, and *Torulopsis* forms blastoconidia only

(Koneman et al.)

36. Which of the following is not characteristic of *Dientamoeba fragilis*?

   A. Easily recognized by its rapid, jerky motility
   B. No known cyst stage, trophozoite shaped like an amoeba
   C. One or two nuclei which have no peripheral chromatin
   D. Flagellate, which is an intestinal pathogen

The answer is A. *D. fragilis* is now classified with the flagellates because of its internal similarities to the trichomonads as demonstrated by electron microscopy. As its name suggests, it usually has two nuclei in the trophozoite form. In addition, it has no known cyst stage. *D. fragilis* moves like an amoeba with a slow, progressive, gliding motion. (Garcia et al.)

37. A thick film has been prepared from a patient suspected of having malaria. It is stained with Wright's stain. Inclusions seen in the patient's erythrocytes are described as blue disks with red nuclei. The infected erythrocytes are generally enlarged and some of them have granules of brownish pigment. Many of the erythrocytes appear to have more than 15 parasites in a single cell. Identify the parasite described.

   A. *Plasmodium falciparum*
   B. *Plasmodium malariae*
   C. *Plasmodium ovale*
   D. *Plasmodium vivax*

The answer is D. *P. vivax* is a *Plasmodium* species that prefers young erythrocytes (reticulocytes), which may be slightly larger than the average red cell on a peripheral smear. The typical appearance of the *Plasmodium* trophozoite on a Wright's-stained smear is the "signet ring," a blue ring with a red nuclear mass. Reddish or brown granules known as Schüffner's dots may be seen in red cells infected in either *P. vivax* or *P. ovale*. *P. vavax* commonly divides to produce a total of 12 to 24 nuclear masses within a single erythrocyte. *P. ovale* usually produces four to 12 merozoites during schizogony. (Finegold et al.)

38. The diagnostic of *Strongyloides stercoralis* infection is the

   A. Egg
   B. Cyst
   C. Larva
   D. Trophozoite

The answer is C. *Strongyloides* does not develop cyst or trophozoite stages. The female lays her eggs in the patient's intestinal mucosa. Ordinarily the eggs hatch in the mucosa and mature into the rhabditiform larvae, which appear in the feces. *Strongyloides* eggs do not appear in the stool except in very severe diarrhea. These eggs resemble the hookworm egg in general size and shape. The two are distinguished by the fact that *Strongyloides* ova are not embryonated when passed. (Finegold et al.; Markell et al.)

39. Trematodes that mature in the lung and produce eggs that appear in the sputum or stool are probably

   A. *Fasciolopsis buski*
   B. *Schistosoma japonicum*
   C. *Paragonimus westermani*
   D. *Clonorchis sinensis*

The answer is C. Although all the parasites listed are flukes capable of infecting humans, only *Paragonimus* consistently invades the lung. *F. buski*, *S. japonicum*, and *C. sinensis* parasitize the intestine, blood vessels, and liver, respectively. (Garcia et al.)

40. A 15-year-old girl was admitted with severe headache and confusion. An examination of her spinal fluid revealed many small, motile amebae. The girl was visiting friends in Georgia and had been swimming and diving in a freshwater pond. The most likely genus and species of the organism is

   A. *Entamoeba histolytica*
   B. *Endolimax nana*
   C. *Iodamoeba bütschlii*
   D. *Naegleria fowleri*

The answer is D. Certain free-living water amebae can cause primary meningo-encephalitis. Fatalities have been reported in the United States, Belgium, Australia, England, and Czechoslovakia. Illness begins with headaches and mild fever, and sometimes, sore throat and rhinitis. While headache and fever increase over the next 3 days, vomiting and neck rigidity develop. Soon the patient becomes disoriented and may lapse into a coma and die. Most case studies to date have occurred following swimming and diving in warm ponds or pools containing water amebae. It is postulated that the amebae gain entrance through the nasal passages, invade along the olfactory nerves, and spread via the subarachnoid space. The ameba most frequently associated with primary amebic meningoen-cephalitis is *Naegleria fowleri*. *Hartmannella* and *Acanthamoeba* have also been reported, rarely, as causative agents. (Finegold et al.; Markell et al.)

41. The causative agent of Q fever is

   A. *Coxiella burnetii*
   B. *Rickettsia typhi (mooseri)*
   C. *Rickettsia rickettsii*
   D. *Rickettsia tsutsugamushi*

The answer is A. Three of the more important rickettsial diseases in the United States are Rocky Mountain spotted fever, Q fever, and murine typhus. *C. burnetii* causes Q fever. *R. mooseri* is the agent of murine typhus. *R. rickettsii* causes Rocky Mountain spotted fever, and *R. tsutsugamushi* causes scrub typhus. (Lennette et al.)

42. Cerebrospinal fluid from a 24-year-old man reveals a high number of mononuclear cells and a negative routine culture for bacteria. Spinal fluid, glucose, and protein values are normal. In addition, the patient has vesicular genital lesions. The most likely etiologic agent is

   A. *Neisseria meningitidis*
   B. Rotavirus
   C. *Chlamydia trachomatis*
   D. Herpes simplex virus

The answer is D. *N. meningitidis* does not cause vesicular lesions, and if infection of the meninges were involved, glucose levels would be below normal. Rotavirus is a common cause of infant diarrhea and is not known to cause skin lesions. *C. trachomatis* genital lesions are characteristically nonvesicular, whereas those caused by herpes simplex virus are vesicular. Herpes simplex genital infection may rarely progress to meningitis, which would result in a mononuclear infiltrate to the CSF but no change in the CSF glucose levels. (Lennette et al.)

43. A 20-year-old man with urethritis who had been treated with penicillin returns to the outpatient clinic the following week. A possible cause of his symptoms is *Chlamydia trachomatis,* which may be confirmed by

    A. Inoculating the specimen onto selective media
    B. Demonstrating glycogen-positive inclusion bodies in the cell culture
    C. Performing a direct Gram stain for gram-negative rods
    D. Performing a blind passage of cells

The answer is B. The recommended technique for in vitro isolation of *C. trachomatis* is tissue culture. Many laboratories use the McCoy cell line. After incubation for 48 to 72 hr, the cell monolayer is stained with iodine. *C. trachomatis*—infected cell cultures are detected by glycogen-positive inclusions. *C. trachomatis* usually cannot be visualized by direct Gram stain. (Lennette et al.)

44. Bacteriophage typing is of greatest value in

    A. Differentiating between the genera *Staphylococcus* and *Micrococcus*
    B. Distinguishing the different species of *Staphylococcus*
    C. Detecting the source of nosocomial infections due to *Staphylococcus aureus*
    D. Determining strains of *Staphylococcus* that have unique susceptibility patterns.

The answer is C. Various strains of staphylococci can be segregated into specific types by identifying a unique marker to trace similar strains. When an outbreak of staphylococcal food poisoning or suspected nosocomial infection occurs, it may be desirable to detect the source of the outbreak. Although a variety of techniques have been used for epidemiologic typing, the established method is bacteriophage typing. This procedure involves comparing patterns of lysis produced by test strains of *S. aureus* to a battery of phages. Distinctive lytic patterns are observed that serve as traces among the various strains of the species. (Lennette et al.)

45. A method of value in the epidemiologic study of outbreaks of infection due to *Pseudomonas aeruginosa* is

    A. Antimicrobic susceptibility testing
    B. Biotyping
    C. Morphologic typing
    D. Pyocin typing

The answer is D. Pyocin typing may be used to trace a source of *P. aeruginosa* in a nosocomial outbreak, although it generally is a reference technique. Antibiograms are usually quite resistant and do not serve to differentiate strains. Similarly, biotyping and morphologic features do not distinguish clearly between strains. Pyocin typing, serotyping, and bacteriophage typing have been used singly and in combination to trace strains of *P. aeruginosa*. (Lennette et al.)

46. Falsely decreased zone diameters on a Kirby-Bauer agar disk diffusion test would most likely result from

   A. An inoculum that is less turbid than a 0.5 MacFarland standard
   B. Use of disks with a higher-than-recommended concentration of antimicrobial
   C. A 2-hr delay in placing the antimicrobial disks on the seeded plate
   D. A 2-hr delay in incubating the plates after the disks have been applied

The answer is C. A 2-hr delay in placing antimicrobial-containing disks on the seeded plate would allow the organism to multiply before the antimicrobial is applied. This factor will result in falsely small zone sizes. Other factors that may cause falsely decreased zone size include the use of Mueller-Hinton agar at a depth of greater than 4 mm, use of deteriorated disks, and an increase in the concentration of calcium or magnesium ions in the agar when testing *Pseudomonas aeruginosa* with the aminoglycosides. The use of a mixed culture may also cause falsely small zones in cases in which one organism is sensitive to a drug, and the other organism is resistant. If the inoculum is too sparse, fewer organisms will result in falsely increased zone diameters. Using antimicrobial disks with higher-than-recommended concentrations of antimicrobials enhances diffusion and allows more organisms to be inhibited. Delaying more than 15 min after disks are applied before incubating plates allows excess prediffusion of antibiotics. These factors result in falsely increased zone diameters. Other factors that may produce falsely large zones include use of Mueller-Hinton agar thinner than 4 mm and too light an inoculum. (Lennette et al.)

47. In interpreting a minimal inhibitory concentration (MIC) by the macrobroth dilution method, you determine that the first test tube that shows visible turbidity has a final dilution factor of 1:32. Since twofold serial dilutions are made from the working stock of 0.256 mg/ml, the MIC for this isolate is

   A. 4 μg/ml
   B. 8 μg/ml
   C. 16μg/ml
   D. 32 μg/ml

The answer is C. Since the MIC end point is the lowest concentration of the antimicrobial at which no visible growth can be detected, the end point in this problem is the 1:16 dilution. To calculate the concentration of antimicrobial at this dilution, divide the stock concentration of 256 μg/ml by the dilution factor of 16. Thus, the MIC is 16 μg/ml. (Lennette et al.)

48. In a synergy study, when drug A, drug B, and drug A + B act singly and in combination on a single population of growing bacteria in vitro as illustrated, the type of killing action signified is

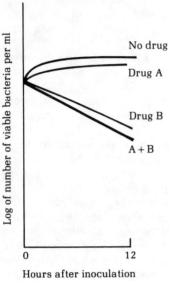

(Source: From J. A. Washington, *Laboratory Procedures in Clinical Microbiology*. New York: Springer, 1981, p. 725)

A. Antagonism
B. Indifference
C. Synergism
D. Not determinable from this representation

The answer is B. Synergy studies test the effect of combinations of antimicrobials on the rate of killing of microbes and may be indicated in the treatment of serious infections. The purpose is to determine if the two drugs in combination are *synergistic* (the effect of the two drugs together is greater than the sum of the effects of either drug alone), *indifferent* (the combined effect does not exceed the sum of the independent effects), or *antagonistic* (the combined drugs are less effective than one of the drugs alone). Examples of the three types of interactions are depicted below. (Washington)

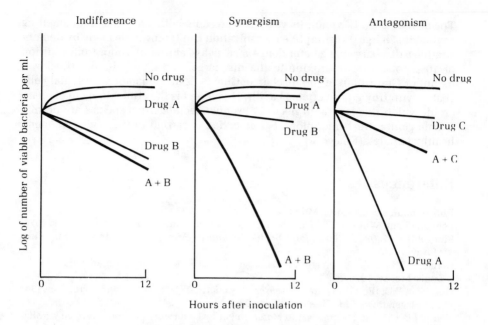

Hours after inoculation

(Source: From J. A. Washington, *Laboratory Procedures in Clinical Microbiology*. New York: Springer, 1981, p. 725)

49. In the Kirby-Bauer agar disk diffusion susceptibility test, a steady decrease in zone diameter of the penicillin disks obtained with the control organism *Staphylococcus aureus*, ATCC 25923, may be due to the fact that the

A. *S. aureus* control strain is too old.
B. Penicillin disks were not stored frozen.
C. pH of the agar is less than 7.2.
D. Mueller-Hinton agar is too thick.

The answer is B. Since only the zones for penicillin are decreasing, a problem with the penicillin disks is probable. Antimicrobial disk cartridges that contain drugs belonging to the penicillin or cephalosporin family should be stored frozen to maintain their potency. A decrease in zone size with the control strain of *S. aureus* and the penicillin disks indicates that the disks are no longer fully potent. This may be due to improper storage conditions. Other factors that cause disk deterioration are humidity and contamination. (Lennette et al.)

50. "Clue cells" seen in a malodorous vaginal discharge are associated with a diagnosis of bacterial vaginosis with

A. *Gardnerella vaginalis*
B. *Haemophilus ducreyi*
C. *Lactobacillus* species
D. *Streptococcus agalactiae*

The answer is A. *G. vaginalis* vaginosis presents with a copious, foul-smelling vaginal discharge. Presumptive identification can typically be made by demonstrating a discharge pH greater than 4.5, a "fishy" amine-like odor from addition of 10% potassium hydroxide to the discharge, and clue cells on direct wet mount or Gram stain of the discharge. Clue cells are squamous epithelial cells coated with tiny gram-variable bacilli. *H. ducreyi* is the etiologic agent of chancroid, which displays with necrotic lesions. *Lactobacillus* species are normal female genital-tract microflora. *S. agalactiae* is carried in the vagina by many healthy females. (Finegold)

References

BBL Manual. Cockeysville, Md.: Becton-Dickinson, 1973.

Fenner, FJ and White, D.O. *Medical Virology* (2nd ed.). New York: Academic Press, 1976.

Finegold, S.M., et al. *Bailey and Scott's Diagnostic Microbiology* (7th ed.). St. Louis: Mosby, 1986.

Garcia, L.S., et. al. *Diagnostic Parasitology: Clinical Laboratory Manual* (2nd ed.). St. Louis: Mosby, 1979.

Hoeprich, P.D. (Ed.). *Infectious Diseases: A Modern Treatise of Infectious Processes* (3rd ed.). Hagerstown, Md.: Harper & Row, 1983.

Henry, J.B. *Clinical Diagnosis and Management by Laboratory Methods* (17th ed.). Philadelphia: Saunders, 1984.

Koneman, E.W., et. al. *Color Atlas and Textbook of Diagnostic Microbiology* (2nd ed.). Philadelphia: Lippencott, 1983.

Lennette, E.H., et. al. *Manual of Clinical Microbiology* (4th ed.). Washington, D.C.: American Society for Microbiology, 1985.

Markell, E.K., et al. *Medical Parasitology* (5th ed.). Philadelphia: Saunders, 1981.

Ross, D.L., et. al. *Textbook of Urinalysis and Body Fluids.* New York: Appleton-Century-Crofts, 1983.

Volk, W.A. *Essentials of Medical Microbiology* (3rd ed.). Philadelphia, Lippincott, 1986.

Washington, J.A. *Laboratory Procedures in Clinical Microbiology.* New York: Springer, 1981.

Laboratory Practice   5

Section Editor
Suzanne Conner, M.A.

Contributors
Ellen R. Bailey
Lois A. Breidenbach
Merry Carter, M.Ed.
Jacqueline Hartfiel, M.S.
Mary Hartke, M.Ed.
Cathy Horton
Richard W. Hubbard, Ph.D.
Frederick W. Law, M.S.
Sandra McLachlan
G. E. Pendergraph, Ph.D.
Tim Porter, M.A.
Lucy Randles, M.A.
Barbara A. Schultz
June Tolin
W. Ard Watson, III, M.S.

CLT Review Questions

1. How should sodium hydroxide burns of the skin be treated?

   A. Flush with copious amounts of water.
   B. Flush with 10% hydrochloric acid and copious amounts of water.
   C. Flush with 5% ammonium hydroxide and copious amounts of water.
   D. Rush the victim to the nearest emergency facility.

The answer is A. For chemical burns of the skin, wash away the chemical with large amounts of water, using a shower or hose as quickly as possible and for at least 5 min. Remove the victim's clothing from the areas involved. (Rose)

2. Which of the following procedures is most basic and effective in preventing the spread of infectious diseases in the hospital environment?

   A. Wearing face masks and gloves in the presence of patients
   B. Wearing laboratory coats in patient rooms
   C. Wearing laboratory coats in the laboratory
   D. Washing hands between each patient contact

The answer is D. It has been said that soap, water, and common sense are the best disinfectants. Although laboratory coats, masks, and gloves have their place and are important in certain situations, the single most effective means of reducing nosocomial infections is frequent and thorough hand washing between patient contacts. (Rose)

3. A clinical laboratory technician determines that a minimum of 85 ml of working reagent is needed for a procedure. To prepare a 1:5 dilution of reagent from a stock solution, one should measure

   A. 15 ml of stock solution and dilute to 85 ml
   B. 20 ml of stock solution and dilute to 100 ml
   C. 25 ml of stock solution and dilute with 125 ml
   D. 30 ml of stock solution and dilute with 125 ml

The answer is B. Dilution usually refers to the volume of concentrate in the total volume of final solution. If 20 ml of the stock are diluted to a total volume of 100 ml, 20 ml/100 ml = $\frac{1}{5}$. (Campbell)

4. Calculate the concentration in millequivalents (mEq) for a solution containing 58.5 mg/dl of NaCL. (Atomic weights: Na = 23; Cl = 35.5)

   A. 1.0 mEq/L
   B. 5.0 mEq/L
   C. 10.0 mEq/L
   D. 20.0 mEq/L

The answer is C.

$$mEq/L = \frac{mg/100\ ml \times 10 \times valence}{atomic\ mass}$$

$$mEq/L = \frac{58.5\ mg/dl \times 10 \times 1}{58.5} = 10\ mEq/L$$

(Campbell)

5. How many grams of sodium hydroxide are required to prepare a 200-ml solution of a 10% (weight per volume) solution? (Atomic weights: Na = 23; O = 16; H = 1)

   A. 4 g
   B. 10 g
   C. 20 g
   D. 40 g

The answer is C.

10% = 10 g/100 ml

X g/200 ml = 10 g/100 ml

100X = 2000

X = 20 g

(Campbell)

6. How much NaCl is needed to make a 0.85% saline solution?

   A. 85 g/L
   B. 0.85 g/L
   C. 8.5 g/L
   D. 850 g/L

The answer is C. A percent solution designates the number of grams of solute per 100 ml of solvent.

8.5 g/L = 0.85 g/100 ml

(Campbell)

7. 11.0 mg/dl of serum calcium is equivalent to which of the following? (Atomic weight of Ca = 40.)

   A. 2.6 mmol/L
   B. 2.75 mmol/L
   C. 2.9 mEq/L
   D. 3.15 mEq/L

The answer is B. Convert the weight per volume to weight per liter of solution. The weight per liter is divided by the atomic weight of the ion being calculated.

11 mg/dl = 110 mg/L

.040 g/L = 1 mmol Ca

$$\frac{110}{.040} = 2.75 \text{ mmol/L}$$

(Campbell)

8. The normality of an unknown HCl solution is 7.2. Calculate the specific gravity of this HCl solution given the assay percentage of HCl (21.6%) and the atomic weight of HCl (36.5).

    A. 1.424
    B. 1.217
    C. 1.19
    D. 1.08

The answer is B. Normality is the number of gram equivalents of solute per liter of solution, and molarity is the number of grams of solute per liter of solution.

Density × 10 × percentage = g/L

7.2 eq/L × 36.5 g/eq = 262.8 g/L

Density × 10 = 21.6 × 262.8

Density = 1.217

(Campbell)

9. What is the correct formula to convert degrees Fahrenheit to degrees centigrade?

    A. ⁵⁄₉(°F + 32)
    B. ⁵⁄₉(°F − 32)
    C. ⁹⁄₅(°F + 32)
    D. ⁹⁄₅(°F − 32)

The answer is B. The centigrade scale is divided into 100 degrees and is the unit in which most scientific study is expressed. (Campbell)

10. How many milliliters of 0.75N HCl would be required to neutralize 280 ml of 1.25N NaOH?

    A. 168
    B. 262.5
    C. 467
    D. 560

The answer is C. The formula used to solve this problem is $N_1 \times V_1 = N_2 \times V_2$.

$(.75N) (X) = (1.25N) (280) = 467$ ml

(Campbell)

11. To properly use a volumetric pipet calibrated "to deliver" (TD), one should

    A. Wipe the outside following delivery of the contents.
    B. Drain the contents but do not blow out.
    C. Rinse out the contents several times.
    D. Drain the contents to the lowest etched mark on the volumetric pipet.

The answer is B. The volumetric pipet is designed to deliver a fixed volume of liquid with the greatest accuracy and precision. The tip of the pipet is tapered to slow the flow of liquid to reduce drainage error. When the liquid has ceased to flow, the tip of the pipet is touched to the inner surface of the container and the residual fluid is allowed to flow out by capillary action. Any remaining liquid should not be blown out. (Tietz)

12. Various blanks may be run during spectrophotometric analysis to correct for absorbance contributed by entities of the test system other than the actual color reaction. Which of the following blanks is used to compensate for absorption of the color of the test sample before reagents are added?

    A. Reagent blank
    B. Water blank
    C. Alcohol blank
    D. Serum blank

The answer is D. A water blank is used when no interfering absorbance is contributed by any part of the test system. A reagent blank is used if there is appreciable absorbance contributed by one or more reagents in the system. Alcohol can be a type of reagent blank. In this instance, a serum blank should be run if the color of the sample itself causes absorption at the wavelength being used. (Henry)

13. What is the total magnification produced when using a 10X ocular lens and a 40X objective lens on a light microscope?

    A. 4,000X
    B. 800X
    C. 400X
    D. Cannot be determined without additional information

The answer is C. Magnification power of a microscope is the product of the enlarging ability of the objective lens and that of the ocular lens. The resolving power of the microscope is provided by the objective lens, and the ocular lens magnifies the image coming from the objectives lens. (Sonnenwirth, et al.)

14. If a technician performing routine microscopic analysis on unstained urine sediment is to have sufficient contrast and resolution to identify important elements, the microscope must be adjusted by

   A. Lowering the condenser and reducing the light
   B. Lowering the condenser and increasing the light
   C. Raising the condenser and reducing the light
   D. Raising the condenser and increasing the light

The answer is A. To have the appropriate "black-white" contrast and sufficient resolution to identify important urine sediment structures in unstained preparations, especially casts, the amount of light must be reduced. For most microscopes this can be done effectively by both lowering the condenser and decreasing the setting on the rheostat. (Sonnenwirth et al.)

15. Which part of the microscope should be adjusted to increase brightness of a microscopic field?

   A. Condenser
   B. Iris diaphragm
   C. Light source rheostat
   D. Prism

The answer is C. Misalignment of the light source and optical axis is probably the most common type of misuse of the microscope. Visible light from the bulb is internally reflected by a mirror into the optical axis of the microscope. This light must be collected and focused on the object on the stage. The condenser is a combination of lenses beneath the stage that focuses the light on the object at an optimal level. The iris diaphragm regulates the diameter of the light field relative to the numerical aperture of the objective lens. Neither the iris diaphragm nor the condenser should be used to control brightness since that would result in a loss of resolution, which is particularly critical at high magnifications. The purpose of the rheostat, normally included in the microscope base, is to control the brightness of illumination. (Sonnenwirth et al.)

16. Applications for employment must conform to

   A. Better Business Bureau guidelines
   B. Clinical Laboratory Improvement Act of 1967 regulations
   C. Title VII of the Civil Rights Act
   D. National Labor Relations Act regulations

The answer is C. An employment application is considered a screening tool to eliminate unqualified people from consideration for employment and must not be discriminatory or have a disparate impact on minorities. Title VII of the Civil Rights Act (1964) guarantees equality to all persons. The act has been amended by the Equal Opportunity Act of 1972, the Pregnancy Discrimination Act of 1978, the Rehabilitation Act of 1973, and the Age Discrimination Employment Act of 1967. (Karni et al.)

17. Which of the following statistics is determined by the formula shown below?

$$\sqrt{\frac{\Sigma\,(X - \overline{X})^2}{n - 1}}$$

    A. Mean
    B. Standard deviation
    C. Variance
    D. Confidence limits

The answer is B. The standard deviation is an attempt to represent a true or reproducible measure of dispersion in quantitative determinations. The first step is to note the amount by which the individual measurements differ from the mean and to calculate the average of these deviations. The deviations are squared to eliminate negative signs. The result to this point is called the *variance*, or the square of deviations. We then take the square root of the variance to convert the statistic to a workable form. The positive square root of the variance is known as the standard deviation. (Henry)

18. If a ground circuit in an instrument wire is *not* complete

    A. The instrument will not work.
    B. Current leakage may cause a shock to the operator.
    C. The fuse or circuit breaker will blow.
    D. A fire will result.

The answer is B. To avoid shocks, all instruments must be grounded. The third wire is provided to drain leakage currents harmlessly to ground. A ground prong should never be cut off because the old receptacle only has two slots. If it is necessary to connect a three-prong plug to a two-slot receptacle, an adapter should be used and the ground wire of the adapter must be securely attached to the retaining screw of the receptacle coverplate to avoid shock. (Sonnenwirth et al.)

19. Which of the following has the highest incidence of infectious risk in the clinical laboratory?

    A. Hepatitis
    B. Infectious mononucleosis
    C. Acquired immunodeficiency syndrome (AIDS)
    D. Rubella

The answer is A. Viral hepatitis is the leading cause of laboratory-acquired infections. The Occupational Safety and Health Administration (OSHA) estimated that approximately 200 health care workers have died of the bloodborne hepatitis B because of occupational exposure between September 1986 and September 1987. Human blood can transmit a number of infectious diseases such as hepatitis and AIDS, and should be treated as a potentially infectious material.

The risk of infection is directly related to the degree of contact with contaminated blood. Infection with the AIDS virus, HIV, has grave consequences but the occurence of hepatitis B is more common and hence the leading infectious risk in the clinical laboratory. (Sonnenwirth et al.; Handsfield et al.)

20. Which of the following represents a diagram of a spectrophotometer?

    A. Hollow cathode—Cuvette—Monochromator—Detector—Readout
    B. Cuvette—Light source—Monochromator—Detector—Readout
    C. Monochromator—Light source—Cuvette—Detector—Readout
    D. Light source—Monochromator—Cuvette—Detector—Readout

The answer is D. The light source is usually a tungsten lamp; monochromators are either a diffraction grating, prism, or filter; cuvettes are made from glass, quartz, or plastic; detectors are barrier-layer cells or photomultiplier tubes; readout devices may be meters, digital devices, or microprocessors. (Tietz)

21. Which of the following instruments is used to measure the speed of a centrifuge?

    A. Volt-ohm-meter (VOM)
    B. Refractometer
    C. Tachometer
    D. Potentiometer

The correct answer is C. An external tachometer of known accuracy should be used to calibrate the speed of a centrifuge; the tachometer should be used to check the speed of the centrifuge at least every 3 months for all speeds at which the centrifuge is routinely used. (Tietz)

22. The wavelengths in the ultraviolet region are

    A. 620 to 700 nm
    B. Over 700 nm
    C. 400 to 450 nm
    D. Below 400 nm

The answer is D. Wavelengths visible to the unaided eye occur at approximately 400 to 700 nm. Ultraviolet light is not visible and occurs at wavelengths below 400 nm. Infrared wavelengths occur above 700 nm. (Tietz)

23. A colorimeter differs from a spectrophotometer in that a colorimeter uses

    A. Precalibrated scales
    B. A constant voltage supply
    C. Filters
    D. A diffraction grating or quartz prism

The answer is C. Photometric instruments have some means of isolating a narrow wavelength range of the spectrum. Those that use filters are called filter photometers or colorimeters and those with a diffraction grating or prism are called spectrophotometers because they produce the entire visible spectrum from which a specific wavelength is isolated. (Tietz)

24. Which of the following wavelengths of light are visible to the unaided eye?

   A. 300 to 700 nm
   B. 200 to 800 nm
   C. 400 to 700 nm
   D. 400 to 900 nm

The answer is C. Only electromagnetic radiation with a wavelength between approximately 400 and 700 nm is visible to the unaided eye. The color of light is determined by its wavelength, with red having the longest wavelength and blue the shortest. (Sonnenwirth et al.)

25. Flammable chemicals such as waste ether and chloroform

   A. May be flushed down the drain with copious amounts of water
   B. May be safely sent to a landfill with the regular trash
   C. Should be incinerated
   D. Should not be used in the clinical laboratory because of the danger

The answer is C. Flammable chemicals can fill the sewer vents with vapors that are a fire hazard. Such flammables should be incinerated or otherwise specially handled by an approved chemical waste hauler. (Sonnenwirth et al.)

26. One nanometer is equal to

   A. 10^{-2} meter
   B. 10^{-6} meter
   C. 10^{-9} meter
   D. 10^{-12} meter

The answer is C. Wavelength of light is the distance between peaks as the light travels in a wavelike manner. This distance is expressed in nanometers (nm). 1 nm = 10^{-9} m. (Tietz)

27. During wavelength calibration of the bench model spectrophotometer with a didymium filter (minimum percent transmittance [%T] at 585 nm), the following data are noted:

585 nm: 52 %T
590 nm: 60 %T
580 nm: 48 %T

Which of the following courses of action would you take?

A. Leave as is; the wavelength calibration is correct.
B. Set the wavelength dial at 585 nm; turn the wavelength calibration screw until minimum %T registers on the scale.
C. Set the wavelength dial at 585 nm; turn the wavelength calibration screw until maximum %T registers on the scale.
D. Adjust the wavelength calibration screw until green light comes through the sample well and attempt the procedure again.

The correct answer is B. The correct procedure to follow is to set minimum %T at 585 nm; the color that should be selected at 585 nm by the monochromator is yellow. The actual minimum %T for didymium may vary, but should be specified on the filter itself. (Tietz)

28. Storage of computer data may be done

A. With magnetic disc or tape
B. On a cathode ray tube (CRT)
C. In the central processing unit (CPU)
D. On a video display terminal (VDT)

The answer is A. Both a CRT and a VDT allow the operator to visualize the data as they are entered. A CPU is the computer chip through which all data flow before they are stored. The principal means of storing data is on magnetic disc or tape. Data retrieval is faster from disc than it is from tape. (McNeely)

29. The following are examples of monochromators used in colorimeters except the

A. Barrier-layer cell
B. Prism
C. Diffraction grating
D. Interference filter

The correct answer is A. A barrier-layer cell is a type of detector found in simple colorimeters, whereas prisms, diffraction gratings (transmittance and reflectance), and interference filters are all examples of monochromators. (Tietz)

30. Chemicals such as sodium hydroxide and sulfuric acid should be labeled

A. Poison
B. Corrosive
C. Biohazard
D. Irritant

The answer is B. Corrosives used in the laboratory are defined as acids or bases that can etch flesh with first-, second-, or third-degree burns 24 hr after contact. Some corrosives destroy live tissue immediately; others cause damage after they have penetrated into deeper tissues. Inhalation of corrosive vapors or ingestion of corrosives causes severe edema and extensive burning of the respiratory tract or mouth and throat. All containers of corrosive acids and bases should be labeled with a CORROSIVE label. Eye, respiratory, and skin protection should be worn when working with corrosives. (Rose)

31. Which of the following has the lowest flashpoint and is therefore the most flammable?

    A. Ether
    B. Isopropyl alcohol
    C. Chloroform
    D. Methanol

The answer is A. The temperature at which a flammable or combustible liquid gives off enough vapor to form an ignitable mixture with air is called the flashpoint of a liquid. Ether has a flashpoint of $-49°F$. (Rose)

32. A patient has a serum calcium level of 11.4 mg/dl. How would this be reported in milliequivalents per liter?

    A. 0.29 mEq/L
    B. 0.57 mEq/L
    C. 2.9 mEq/L
    D. 5.7 mEq/L

The correct answer is D. To convert milligrams per deciliter to milliequivalents per liter, you must use the following formula:

$$mEq/L = \frac{mg/dl \times 10}{Equivalent\ mass}$$

Equivalents per liter is determined by dividing grams per liter by equivalent mass, so milliequivalents per liter would be determined by dividing milligrams per liter by equivalent mass. To convert milligrams per deciliter to milligrams per liter multiply by 10. The equivalent mass of calcium is calculated by dividing its atomic mass (40) by its ionic charge or valence (2). Thus

$$mEq/L = \frac{11.4\ mg/dl \times 10}{20} = 5.7\ mEq/L$$

(Campbell)

33. Which of the following should be performed to determine the optimal wavelength at which to measure the absorbance of a colored solution?

    A. Calibration curve
    B. Wavelength calibration
    C. Spectral transmittance curve
    D. Molar absorptivity calculation

The answer is C. When various wavelengths are plotted vs. %T, a spectral transmittance curve will result which will peak at the wavelength where greatest absorbance or least transmittance occurs. This process can be used to determine the optimal wavelength of light to use for the analysis. This results in improved specificity, sensitivity and linearity of spectrophotometric measurement. (Tietz)

34. Which of the following does the most to minimize aerosol production during centrifugation?

   A. Using a refrigerated centrifuge
   B. Using centrifuge tubes with tapered bottoms
   C. Selecting centrifuge tube sizes that will fit securely into the centrifuge rack
   D. Covering the centrifuge tube with Parafilm or closing with a well-fitting stopper

The correct answer is D. Specimen collection tubes should be left stoppered for centrifugation; if need arises to centrifuge an unstoppered tube, it should be covered with Parafilm or fitted snugly with a stopper. (Tietz)

35. From the following data, calculate the concentration of the analyte in a serum sample read at 560 nm.

   Absorbance of the unknown sample =   0.325
   Absorbance of a 200-mg/dl standard =   0.460

   A. 283 mg/dl
   B. 141 mg/dl
   C. 130 mg/dl
   D. 14.1 mg/dl

The answer is B. Beer's law states that concentration (conc) is directly proportional to absorbance (abs) if the analysis is linear. The calculation is as follows:

$$\frac{\text{abs unknown}}{\text{conc unknown}} = \frac{\text{abs standard}}{\text{conc standard}}$$

$$\frac{0.325}{x} = \frac{0.460}{200} = 141 \text{ mg/dl}$$

(Henry)

36. A serial dilution is set up by pipetting 0.1 ml serum into 0.9 ml saline in tube 1, and serially transferring 0.5 ml through tubes 2, 3, 4, and 5, each of which contains 0.5 ml saline. What is the dilution in tube 5?

   A. 1:16
   B. 1:80
   C. 1:128
   D. 1:160

The correct answer is D. The dilution in tube 1 is 1:10 (1 part serum to 10 parts total solution). Each serial transfer creates an additional 1:2 dilution (5 parts transferred solution to 10 parts new total solution). To determine the dilution of serum saline at any point in the serial dilution, multiply the dilutions made in each tube. To solve this problem, multiply the dilutions made in all five tubes:

Tube No.									Total
$\dfrac{1}{10}$	$\times$	$\dfrac{1}{2}$	$\times$	$\dfrac{1}{2}$	$\times$	$\dfrac{1}{2}$	$\times$	$\dfrac{1}{2}$	$=$ $\dfrac{1}{160}$

(Campbell)

37. If in performing an analysis, the sample reading on a spectrophotometer is more than 90 %T, one should then

   A. Change the wavelength.
   B. Dilute the sample and repeat the test.
   C. Double the sample size and repeat the test.
   D. Choose another method of analysis.

The answer is C. A spectrophotometer reading above 90 %T and below 10 %T indicates loss of sensitivity in the analysis. If the analyte is present in such low concentration to give a reading above 90 %T, the analysis can be repeated using double the amount of specimen and the result divided by 2 to derive the final concentration. (Tietz)

38. A 4.0-mg/dl creatinine standard is needed. To prepare 100 ml of the working standard, how much stock standard of 1 mg/ml creatinine is needed?

   A. 0.1 ml
   B. 0.4 ml
   C. 4 ml
   D. 40 ml

The correct answer is C.

To solve this problem, use the formula:

$Volume_1 \times concentration_1 = Volume_2 \times concentration_2$

where volume$_1$ and concentration$_1$ represent the stock standard and volume$_2$ and concentration$_2$ represent the working standard. Units of concentration must be the same between the stock and working standards, so 1 mg/ml should be expressed as 100 mg/dl to be consistent with the working standard.

$V_1 \times 100$ mg/dl $= 100$ ml $\times 4$ mg/dl

$$V_1 = \frac{100 \text{ ml} \times 4 \text{ mg/dl}}{100 \text{ mg/dl}}$$

(Tietz)

39. A pipet should be wiped off

   A. Before lowering the meniscus to the calibration mark
   B. After lowering the meniscus to the calibration mark
   C. Never if it is a volumetric pipet
   D. Only if it is a TC (to contain) pipet

The answer is A. The pipet should be loaded, wiped, held vertically, then emptied until the meniscus touches the calibration mark. This applies to serologic, volumetric, and TC pipets. (Henry)

40. A laboratory fire ignited by faulty wiring in a chemistry analyzer and partially fueled by surrounding paper products is classified as:

   A. Class B
   B. Class C
   C. Class A and B
   D. Class A and C

The correct selection is D. Paper and other ordinary combustibles constitute a class A fire when ignited, and the burning-energized electric equipment characterizes a class C fire. The situation described above is a combination class A and C fire. (Rose)

41. Which of the following precautions must be observed when working with corrosive materials in the laboratory?

   A. Work in a class II biosafety cabinet.
   B. Wear gloves and goggles.
   C. Wear face protection and shoe covers.
   D. Put corrosive material in container and add water.

The answer is B. When handling corrosive solutions, laboratory personnel should wear goggles or a face mask, do any stirring or mixing in a fume hood, avoid wearing contact lenses, and wear protective gloves. (Rose)

42. Which of the following has been prohibited from use on anything other than a temporary basis in the clinical laboratory?

   A. Power strips
   B. Portable floor fans
   C. Extension cords
   D. Multi-outlet boxes

The correct selection is C. In 1980, the National Committee for Clinical Laboratory Standards (NCCLS) standard on power requirements for clinical laboratories prohibited the use of extension cords except under certain temporary conditions. In such cases, cords must be less than 12 feet long, single-outlet, at least 16 AWG wire, and UL-approved. (Tietz)

43. When using cobalt chloride as an indicator of the water absorption capacity of a desiccant, the desiccant should be

    A. Changed when it turns blue
    B. Handled with care because cobalt chloride is a carcinogen
    C. Kept in the dark
    D. Changed when it turns pink

The answer is D. A common desiccant is calcium chloride treated with cobalt chloride (Drierite). Cobalt chloride turns pink as water-absorbing capacity is exhausted. Cobalt chloride is neither a carcinogen nor destroyed by sunlight. (Sonnenwirth et al.)

44. On linear coordinate graph paper, using the ordinate for absorbance and the abscissa for concentration, a straight line through the origin and three plotted standards indicates all of the following *except*

    A. The concentration of the standard vs. the absorbance of the standards is linear.
    B. The concentration of the standard vs. the %T is linear.
    C. The test complies with Beer's law.
    D. The concentration of the standard vs. the log %T is an inverse relationship.

The correct answer is B. The standard curve described demonstrates Beer's law; i.e., the concentration is directly proportional to absorbance. Concentration is also inversely proportional to the logarithm of %T. The concentration of the standard does not have a linear relationship with %T. (Tietz)

45. The function of a condenser on a microscope is to

    A. Regulate the amount of light passing through the objective
    B. Magnify the image
    C. Reverse the image
    D. Project and center the light through the specimen and objective lens

The answer is D. The condenser is a combination of lenses beneath the stage that focuses the light on the specimen and also provides a cone of light sufficient for the numerical aperture (NA) of the objective lens. The condenser should not be used to control brightness as it will result in loss of resolution. Brightness should be controlled by the rheostat on the light source. (Sonnenwirth et al.)

46. Beer's law can be expressed as:

   A. $C\ unk = \dfrac{abs\ std \times C\ std}{abs\ unk}$
   B. Abs = log %T
   C. Abs = 2 − log %T
   D. Abs = 100 − %T

where c = concentration; abs = absorbance; std = standard; unk = un-known; and %T = percent transmittance.

The answer is C. According to Beer's law, absorbance is directly proportional to the concentration and inversely proportional to the logarithm of transmittance. Since the log 100 = 2, the formula is A = 2 − log %T. (Henry)

47. Beer's law states that the concentration of a substance is

   A. Directly proportional to the amount of light absorbed
   B. Inversely proportional to the concentration
   C. Proportional to the logarithm of the transmitted light
   D. Proportional to the square root of the concentration

The answer is A. The light absorption is proportional to the number of mole-cules of absorbing substance through which the light passes. If the absorbing substance is dissolved in a transparent medium, the absorbtion of the solution is proportional to its molecular concentration. (Henry)

48. The term *computer software* consists of

   A. The program and operating system
   B. Memory, program, and printout
   C. CPU and program
   D. All the data stored in volatile memory

The answer is A. Software is the part of the computer system you cannot touch. Software gives the computer instructions as to how to carry out different tasks. It consists of programs and the operating system. (McNeely)

49. When a blue filter is placed in the path of a white light source, the filter will

   A. Transmit wavelengths other than blue
   B. Transmit the red wavelengths
   C. Absorb only the blue wavelengths
   D. Absorb wavelengths other than blue

The answer is D. A solution will appear blue because it transmits wavelengths in the blue portion of the spectrum and absorbs light of other wavelengths. (Tietz)

50. A control has a mean of 5.5 with a standard deviation of 0.5. If the laboratory is using a 95% confidence interval, the control values must fall between

A. 4.5 to 6.5
B. 5.0 to 6.0
C. 4.0 to 7.0
D. 5.0 to 6.5

The answer is A. A confidence limit or confidence interval of 95% is equal to the mean plus or minus 2 SDs. In this case it is equal to 5.5 ± 1 or 4.5 to 6.5. (Tietz)

CLS Review Questions

1. Chemicals exist in varying degrees of purity. For quantitative measurements and preparation of accurate standard solutions, it is important to use pure chemicals labeled as

A. Technical grade
B. Reagent grade
C. Purified
D. *United States Pharmacopeia (USP)*

The answer is B. For quantitative measurements and preparation of accurate standard solutions, it is important to use pure chemicals and to identify exact amounts of compounds or elements desired, as well as amount of contaminants. The use of *reagent-grade* chemicals, although more expensive than using less pure grades of chemicals, is essential to accuracy. Because several grades of chemicals are available, an awareness of the terms used widely is necessary. For the most highly purified chemicals, either *reagent grade, analytical grade,* or *ACS* (for having met standards of purity established by the American Chemical Society) should appear on the label or in the catalogue. Less pure chemicals are referred to as *purified* and *technical.* (Henry)

2. Which of the following statements does *not* apply to dry chemical fire extinguishers?

A. They can be used on flammable liquid fires involving live electric equipment.
B. They can be used on class A, B, and C fires.
C. They can be used on fires in which a re-ignition source is present.
D. They contain ingredients that are nontoxic.

The answer is C. Dry chemical fire extinguishers can be used on flammable liquid fires and fires involving live electricity (classes B and C) because the chemical does not conduct electricity. Because it rapidly extinguishes fire, dry chemical is also often used on fires involving combustible materials (class A). However, because the use of a dry chemical does not produce a permanently inert atmosphere above the fire surface, if there is any possibility of re-ignition, such as from hot surfaces or smoldering embers, additional appropriate extinguishing agents such as foam must be used. (Rose)

3. Monitoring the work area in which radioactive substances such as iodine 125 and carbon 14 are handled is an important aspect of maintaining safe working conditions. Such monitoring may be performed in a number of ways, the most sensitive of which is

   A. Visual examination of the work area
   B. Survey of the work area with a thin-window Geiger-Müller counter
   C. Wipe-sample analysis of the work area
   D. Survey of the work area with a general, all-purpose, Geiger-Müller counter

The answer is C. The wipe-sample analysis is much more sensitive than the survey meter for most radionuclides. A Geiger-Muller counter, even with a thin window, is not sensitive enough to register low-level beta emissions such as those from carbon 14 and tritium. A laboratory using both gamma and beta emitters should be monitored by wipe-testing the work area, with the sample filters counted in a liquid scintillation counter. (Miller)

4. The most environmentally acceptable method for disposal of most chemical waste products is

   A. Burial
   B. Disposal to sewer system
   C. Incineration
   D. Evaporation

The answer is C. Incineration is currently the most acceptable method for chemical waste disposal. The process of combustion of organic material with excess oxygen, high temperatures, and extended time results in the degradation of the original compound to its elemental form. The use of landfill or burial for disposal can lead to a later contamination of the environment with the waste material. Laboratories using this method must comply with all applicable local, state, and federal regulations. Laboratories must also comply with all appropriate regulations if water-soluble chemicals are disposed of into the public sewer systems. Evaporation, under controlled conditions, is a useful technique only for a limited number of volatile substances. (Karni et al.)

5. A 200-mg/dl solution was diluted 1:10. This diluted solution was then additionally diluted 1:5. What is the concentration of the final solution?

   A. 2 mg/dl
   B. 4 mg/dl
   C. 20 mg/dl
   D. 40 mg/dl

The answer is B. To calculate final dilutions, multiply the original concentration by the dilution, expressed as a fraction.

200 mg × $\frac{1}{10}$ × $\frac{1}{5}$ = 4 mg/dl

(Campbell)

6. What is the molarity of an unknown HCl solution that has a specific gravity of 1.10 and an assay percentage of 18.5%? (Atomic weight: HCl = 36.5)

   A. 5.6 M
   B. 6.0 M
   C. 6.3 M
   D. 6.6 M

The answer is A. To solve this problem, it is necessary to convert the density and percentage strength of the strong acid to grams per liter (g/L) and then to molarity.

Density × 10 × percentage = g/L

Molarity = No. of grams of solute per liter of solution

therefore

1.10 × 10 × 18.5 = 203.5 g/L × 1 mole/36.5 g = 5.6 M

(Campbell)

7. A method requires the use of an 8% (weight per volume) solution of NaOH. The available solutions are labeled 1N, 2N, 2.5N, and 10N. Which solution is equivalent to 8% NaOH? (Atomic weights: Na = 23; O = 16; H = 1)

   A. 1N
   B. 2N
   C. 2.5N
   D. 10N

The answer is B. The normality of a solution is equal to the number of gram equivalents of solute per liter of solution or the number of milligram equivalents (mEq) of solute per milliliter of solution.

mEq/L = (mg/100 ml) × 10 × valence/atomic mass

8% (w/v) = 8 g/100 ml or 8,000 mg/100 ml

mEq/L = (8,000 mg) × 10 × valence/40 = 80,000/40 = 2,000

N = 2,000 mEq/L/1,000 ml = 2N

8. Quartz or plastic cuvettes of optical quality should be used when performing spectrophotometric assays in the ultraviolet (UV) region (i.e., less than 340 nm of the spectrum) because the usual borosilicate glass

   A. Refracts light at 340 nm
   B. Contributes to light scatter at 340 nm
   C. Absorbs light at 340 nm
   D. Emits light of a different wavelength

The answer is C. Regular glass cuvettes made of borosilicate glass should not be used for UV determinations because this material absorbs some of the incident light at these wavelengths, resulting in optical densities that are falsely elevated. (Henry)

9. Which of the following best describes the relation of nephelometry to turbidimetry?

   A. Nephelometry measures the amount of light absorbed by particles in solution, and turbidimetry measures the amount of light transmitted through a solution.
   B. Nephelometry directly measures the amount of light scattered by particles in solution, and turbidimetry measures the decrease in incident-light intensity.
   C. Nephelometry measures the amount of light emitted by particles in solution, and turbidimetry measures the amount of light reflected by particles in solution.
   D. Nephelometry measures the amount of light transmitted, and turbidimetry measures the amount of light absorbed.

The answer is B. Turbidimetry is the measurement of the cloudiness of a solution due to the number of particles suspended in solution. It is the decrease in the amount of incident light that is transmitted through the sample that is actually measured. Nephelometry measures directly the amount of light that is scattered or reflected, rather than absorbed, by the particles in suspension. (Henry)

10. Which of the following statements best describes the principle of dark-field microscopy?

   A. Transparent objects are rendered visible by changing the amplitudes of light waves as they pass through the objects under study.
   B. Selective absorption produces a visible image because specimen detail appears as differences in color to which the eye is sensitive.
   C. Light passes through the specimen at an angle, is diffracted, and enters the objective lens, producing a bright image.
   D. A visible image is produced by the use of magnetic fields, making possible greater magnification and resolution.

The answer is C. In dark-field microscopy an opaque disk built into the condenser allows only peripheral rays of light to enter the condenser. These rays pass through the specimen at an angle such that the field appears unilluminated. Any particles in the field will diffract the light and appear bright against a darkened background. Dark-field microscopy is useful in visualizing bacterial flagella and spirochetes, which are poorly defined by bright-field and phase-contrast microscopy. (Sonnenworth et al.)

11. To obtain better separation of liquid and solid components by centrifugation,

    A. Increase the speed of the head.
    B. Decrease the radius of the circle inscribed by the revolving head.
    C. Increase the length of the tube containing the specimen.
    D. Reduce the number of specimens in the centrifuge.

The answer is A. The relative centrifugal force (rcf) is calculated using the following formula:

rcf = 0.00001118 $\times$ r $\times$ N^2

  r = radius of centrifuge head in centimeters
  N = speed in rpm

Thus, rcf can be increased by increasing the speed or the radius of the head. (Henry)

12. Which of the following statements represents the best definition of *alternating current?*

    A. Current that changes direction and value
    B. Current that can change direction, but has a fixed voltage
    C. Current that flows in the same direction, but whose voltage can be altered
    D. Current produced by an alternate power source, such as an electrochemical cell

The answer is A. An *alternating current* is a current that periodically changes direction and value. A direct current always flows in the same direction at some fixed voltage and is produced by an electrochemical cell or battery. (Henry)

13. Ensuring reliability of all steps of a laboratory procedure requires

    A. Use of a serum standard
    B. Incorporation of preanalyzed control material
    C. Duplicate patient testing
    D. Use of a primary standard

The answer is B. The reliability of laboratory procedures is best ensured by incorporating a preanalyzed control in the run of patient specimens. In this way, all steps of the procedure and all variations therein are monitored through acceptance or rejection of the value of the preanalyzed control for the test. Standards may not be subject to all of the same test conditions as the unknowns, whereas the control material would be treated as an unknown. If the test result for the control falls within the preestablished acceptable limits of variation around the mean, the accuracy and precision, and consequently the reliability, of the entire test procedure is ensured. (Tietz)

14. A hematology laboratory in a hospital has determined that the abnormal low RBC control has a mean value of 3.12 million red cells per mm³. The 95% confidence limits include red cell count values from $3.06 \times 10^3/mm^3$ to $3.18 \times 10^6/mm^3$. One standard deviation for this control is equal to

   A. $0.01 \times 10^6/mm^3$
   B. $0.02 \times 10^6/mm^3$
   C. $0.03 \times 10^6/mm^3$
   D. $0.04 \times 10^6/mm^3$

The answer is C. Random errors occur in all laboratory measurements, creating the need for establishing acceptable ranges. When sufficient determinations are made, the distribution of values should follow the gaussian curve of normal distribution. Approximately 68% of the results should fall within 1 SD and 95% within 2 SDs. In the above situation, the laboratory personnel are confident that they can expect their low abnormal RBC control to fall between $3.06 \times 10^6/mm^3$ and $3.18 \times 10^6/mm^3$, 95% of the time. One SD is determined by subtracting the mean, 3.12, from the upper confidence limit, 3.18, and dividing by 2 to equal 0.03. (Henry)

15. In a normal distribution of results, the mean value ± 2 SDs will exclude

   A. 55% of the population
   B. 32% of the population
   C. 5% of the population
   D. 1% of the population

The answer is C. In a normal frequency curve, ± 2 SDs *includes* 95% of the population; therefore, 5% are excluded. (Henry)

16. If a test has a specificity of 98%, it results in approximately

   A. 98% false positives
   B. 98% false negatives
   C. 2% false positives
   D. 2% false negatives

The answer is C. The index of specificity can be calculated using the following formula:

$$\text{Index of specificity} = \frac{\text{true negatives} - \text{false positives}}{\text{true negatives}} \times 100$$

Therefore, the index of specificity reflects the degree of false positive and true negative results that would be expected from a normal population. A highly specific test produces a low incidence of false positive and a high incidence of true positive results. A test with low specificity produces a high incidence of false positive and a low incidence of true positive results. (Henry)

17. The coefficient of variation is the

    A. Square root of the variance from the mean
    B. Standard deviation expressed as a percentage of the mean
    C. Sum of the squared differences from the mean
    D. Confidence interval of the mean

The answer is B. The coefficient of variation (CV), or relative standard deviation, is a statistical tool used to compare variability in nonidentical data sets. To do this, the variability in each data set must be expressed as a relative rather than absolute measure. This is accomplished for each data set by expressing the standard deviation as a percentage of the mean:

$$CV = \frac{SD}{\overline{X}} (100)$$

The CV of each data set allows comparison of two or more test methods, laboratories, or specimen sets. (Campbell)

18. A new method of glucose testing is compared to an accepted reference method by running split samples from 40 patients by each method. The *least squares regression analysis* is calculated. The type of error indicated by an upward shift of the line that does not intersect the origin is a

    A. Constant error
    B. Proportional error
    C. Random error
    D. Systematic error

The answer is A. In the comparison of methods experiment, a plot of data in which there are no analytic errors shows that all the points fall on a straight line that has a 45-degree angle and intersects the origin. Adding 2 mg/dl to the original values, simulating a constant type of systematic analytic error, results in a line that shifts upward by an amount that is constant throughout the range of the graph. The angle of the line is still 45 degrees, but the line does not intersect the origin. (Henry)

19. Comparison of a new test method with a known comparative method is reflected in the solid line of the graph below. The analytic error is

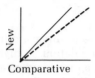

Comparative

    A. Constant
    B. Proportional
    C. Random
    D. Combined and constant and proportional

The answer is B. Ideally, comparison of values obtained by simultaneous testing of a "new" method with an "old" method would result in a straight line graph with a slope of 1.0. When this does not occur, however, the graph is evaluated with respect to analytic error. Proportional error is shown in this graph because it illustrates that the amount of bias is increasing in direct proportion to the concentration of the analyte in the specimen. Constant error would be represented by an operational line parallel to the ideal operational line, and random error would be illustrated by dispersion of data points above and below the ideal operational line. (Henry)

20. A new method for testing an analyte is compared to an accepted reference method by running split samples from 40 patients by each method. The best statistical method for determining whether a significant difference exists between the means of the two methods is

    A. Correlation coefficient
    B. F test
    C. Least squares regression analysis
    D. t test

The answer is D. Statistical tests such as the t test and F test are often used to determine whether a difference exists between the two quantities that are estimates of performance parameters such as the mean (t test) and the variance (F test). The correlation coefficient is a statistic that estimates the degree of association between two variables; a value of 1.0 indicates perfect association. The correlation coefficient is of little value in estimating the analytic errors in the comparison of methods experiment. It is sensitive only to random error and also depends on the range of concentrations studied. The least squares regression analysis is used for estimating the best linear relation between two variables. These statistics provide information about the constant, proportional, and random error between methods. (Weisbrot)

21. Evaluation of random error in a new test method is best accomplished by

  A. Comparison of coefficients of variation for new method and method in use
  B. Replication of determinations on a single sample
  C. Single determinations on an aliquoted specimen for 30 days
  D. Repetition of one complete patient run

The answer is B. Imprecision in laboratory data may be due to any of several factors. To determine the amount of variability *inherent* in the new method, testing should be designed to exclude other factors that may cause unavoidable variability. For this reason replicate analyses on a single sample are recommended to eliminate factors such as day-to-day variability, technologist variability, and reagent variability. (Henry)

22. In the performance of method evaluation experiments, replication experiments should be conducted

  A. Using different test samples in one analytic run over a period of 1 day
  B. Using one test sample in one analytic run over a period of 30 days
  C. To estimate the proportional analytic error
  D. To estimate systematic errors arising when particular materials are added to the sample

The answer is B. A replication experiment estimates the random error that may be caused by factors such as the lack of stability of an instrument, temperature, reagents, or standards or lack of reproducibility in the pipetting, timing, mixing, heating, or analytic technique. The experiment is performed by analyzing several test samples that are aliquots of a single material, such as a control solution. An estimate of day-to-day random error is obtained by analyzing the test samples in several analytic runs that occur on different days. This estimate provides the most realistic estimate of the random error expected in routine operation. (Bruce)

23. The term that means reproducibility among replicate determinations of a sample is

  A. Accuracy
  B. Precision
  C. Reliability
  D. Standard deviation

The answer is B. *Precision* refers to the magnitude of the random errors and the reproducibility of the measurements. The precision of a clinical method is measured by its variance or standard deviation. The smaller the variance, the greater the precision, and if two methods are being compared, the method with the smaller variance is more precise. (Weisbrot)

24. The specificity of a test method is determined by the

    A. Percentage of positive tests in patients who have the disease
    B. Percentage of negative tests in people who do not have the disease
    C. Number of positive tests when the substance being measured is present in low concentration
    D. Ratio of true positives to true negatives

The answer is B. The term *sensitivity* refers to the ability of a test to detect an abnormal state (true positive); the term *specificity* indicates the ability of a test to obtain normal results in nondiseased (true negative) populations. (Henry)

25. A commercial pregnancy test is being evaluated for use in the laboratory as a screening test. Reactions with various urine samples tested are as follows:

Urine Tested	No. Tested	Percent Positive
Pregnant women	100	98
Nonpregnant women	50	6
Men	50	8
Menopausal women	40	15
Ectopic pregnancy	20	15

Which of the following statements is correct?

    A. This appears to be an excellent method for screening patients with ectopic pregnancy because it is highly specific.
    B. This method is not suitable for pregnancy screening because it is too specific.
    C. This method is not suitable for pregnancy screening because it is too sensitive.
    D. This appears to be an excellent method for screening pregnant women because it is highly sensitive.

The answer is D. *Sensitivity* indicates the frequency of positive test results in patients with a particular disease, expressed as a percentage. *Specificity* indicates the frequency of negative test results in patients without the disease, also expressed as a percentage. Most tests are not both highly specific and highly sensitive. Screening tests are expected to have a high degree of sensitivity but are not required to have a high degree of specificity. Since there is a high incidence of positive tests results in patients with normal pregnancy, one cannot conclude that this test is highly specific for ectopic pregnancy only. Therefore, this test would be excellent as a pregnancy screening test but poor as a confirmatory test for ectopic pregnancy. (Sonnenwirth et al.)

26. The "backbone" of any quality control program is primarily

    A. Efficiency
    B. Documentation

C. Proficiency testing
D. Accuracy

The answer is B. The ability to prove that various laboratory tests are accurate and have been repeatedly checked requires documentation that is periodically reviewed in an organized manner. (Henry)

27. What is the effect of allowing a computer disc to come into contact with a magnetic field?

A. The signal is weakened.
B. The data may get mixed up.
C. The data may be erased.
D. No effect; discs are now coated with an antimagnetic spray.

The answer is C. Data are put on discs by arranging the oxide coating in a pattern. When this oxide is disrupted by a magnetic field, the pattern is destroyed and the data may be erased. (McNeely)

28. Careful examination of workload tallies does *not* assist in assessing

A. Productivity
B. Staffing needs
C. Instrument downtime
D. Time needed per test

The answer is C. Workload tallies are sums of raw counts of patient specimen tests, standards, controls, and repeats performed daily in a specific laboratory section for all methods, both manual and automated. From these tallies or workload figures, the need for manpower on certain days, months, and/or shifts can be seen. Decreased workload for a day or short period may reflect instrument malfunction, but the actual hours of downtime cannot be determined because they are not recorded on the workload recording sheets. (Karni et al.)

29. Using the College of American Pathologists (CAP) workload recording system, the unit value assigned to a procedure includes the time for

A. Quality control
B. Specimen processing
C. Specimen collection
D. Repeats

The answer is B. Specimen collection is assigned its own unit value. Quality control time is counted separately and given the same value as specimen processing. Repeats are counted individually because they are performed only when necessary rather than routinely. Specimen processing is the correct answer because it is included in the time-motion study performed to establish the unit value. (Karni et al.)

30. Which of the following tests is *not* included in the raw count of patient specimens for a workload recording system?

    A. Control
    B. Repeat
    C. Replicate
    D. Standard

The answer is C. A replicate test is a test routinely performed in a specific method such as coagulation tests. Since replicate tests are included in the time studies required to establish appropriate unit values, they are part of the unit value and are not counted. Quality control and standard tests are counted and given the same unit values as the patient specimens. Quality control and standard tests do not involve processing a requisition or reporting, but compensatory time is necessary for the recording and statistical aspects of the testing. A repeat test is a test performed to solve a problem that arises when testing a patient specimen. For a repeat test to be counted, the specimen must be retested or analyzed, patient and test data properly handled, and test results recorded. Initial preparation, which includes accession and processing of the specimen, is not included in the definition of a repeat test. (Karni et al.)

36. The chief administrative officer holds the title of president of a large inner city hospital that is governed by a voluntary board of directors composed of community leaders. The hospital revenue continually exceeded its expenses by 5% each year. According to the Internal Revenue Service (IRS) this hospital is a

    A. "For-profit" institution because its income has continually exceeded its expenses
    B. "Not-for-profit" institution because its board of directors is not paid
    C. "For-profit" institution because the chief administrative officer is considered a president
    D. "Not-for-profit" institution because it is located in an inner city area

The answer is B. The profit or nonprofit status of an institution or corporation depends on whether or not net profits are realized by the institution. Reasonable profits are expected and necessary for an organization to survive inflationary trends and provide for improved services. Criteria for nonprofit status under IRS codes are:

1. No private individual(s) benefit from net earnings of the organization.
2. The corporation must operate exclusively for religious, charitable, safety, or educational purposes.
3. The organization cannot refuse services to those unable to pay if the organization is financially able to provide those services without compensation.
4. The use of facilities cannot be restricted to a particular group of physicians and surgeons.
5. The organization cannot loan any money without receiving interest and without security.

6. An employee may not be paid above levels considered acceptable for reimbursement of that individual's services.
7. Investments made and assets sold by the organization must be done with acceptable financial benefit. (Karni et al.)

32. Which federal law removed the exemption of nonprofit hospitals from engaging in collective bargaining with employees?

 A. Occupational Safety and Health Act of 1970
 B. Clinical Laboratory Improvement Act of 1967
 C. Amendment to National Labor Relations Act, 1974
 D. Amendment to Federal Labor Standards Act, 1963

The answer is C. Amendments in 1974 to the National Labor Relations Act (NLRA) removed the previous exemption of nonprofit hospitals that prevented employees from engaging in collective bargaining activities. Employees in independent and physicians' office laboratories also have the right to engage in collective bargaining activities if the laboratory brings in a certain amount of revenue. The Fair Labor Standards Act (FLSA) establishes minimum wages, maximum hours, and certain working conditions. The 1963 amendment to the FLSA eliminates sex-biased wage differentials. (Karni et al.)

33. The regulations from the Clinical Laboratory Improvement Act of 1967 apply to

 A. All clinical laboratories in the United States
 B. Hospital laboratories only
 C. Laboratories engaged in interstate commerce only
 D. Independent laboratories only

The answer is C. The Clinical Laboratory Improvement Act of 1967 applies to any laboratory engaged in interstate commerce (i.e., receiving specimens from other states). The regulations require specific personnel, quality control standards, participation in approved proficiency testing programs, and site inspections. A laboratory found to be in compliance with the regulations receives a license. (Karni et al.)

34. Which of the following theorists worked with the concept that unsatisfied needs are important motivators?

 A. Hawthorne
 B. Herzberg
 C. McGregor
 D. Maslow

The answer is D. According to Maslow, physiologic, safety, security, and social needs are primary needs, which must be satisfied before people are motivated to pursue the secondary needs of esteem and self-actualization. A satisfied need is not a motivator; insufficient satisfaction may cause increased motivation. (Karni et al.)

35. Which of the following must be done before a job description can be written?

    A. Check with other departments in the institution to see if they have similar jobs.
    B. Establish a salary range.
    C. Perform a job analysis.
    D. Establish performance standards.

The answer is C. Each job in an institution must be analyzed for tasks and responsibilities before a job description is written. Standards needed for successful performance of the tasks (performance standards) are established through job analysis. Job analysis is accomplished by observation, interviewing and completion of questionnaires by employees. (Karni et al.)

36. A device that allows computers to communicate via phone lines is a

    A. Modem
    B. CPU
    C. RAM
    D. ROM

The answer is A. A modem (short for modulating-demodulating) is a device that is wired into the telephone line instead of using an acoustic coupler with a handset. The speed at which a computer communicates over the phone lines is measured in bauds (bits audio). Most modems operate at 1200 bauds, or 120 characters per second. (Henry)

37. The computer term used for capturing data from instruments and processing them without delay is

    A. Time-sharing
    B. Batch-processing
    C. Real time
    D. Distributed processing

The answer is C. Real time means that the computer receives the information as it comes from the instrument analyzing the substance and processes it for immediate retrieval. (Henry)

38. Which of the following is essential in stating the conditions of centrifugation in a procedure?

    A. Revolutions per minute (rpm)
    B. Voltage output of centrifuge
    C. Relative centrifugal force (rcf)
    D. Angle of centrifuge head

The answer is C. Conditions for centrifugation should specify both the time and the rcf. The rcf is a function of the radius between the axis of rotation and the center of the centrifuge tube and the number of revolutions per minute.

$$rcf = 0.00001118 \times radius \times rpm^2$$

(Campbell)

39. A laboratory section performs 25 determinations of a specific analyte. The CAP unit value for the procedure is 9.0. Which of the following is correct?

A. The total workload is 225.
B. The work unit is 25.
C. The raw count is 9.0.
D. The total workload is 25.

The answer is A. A work unit is the average technical, clerical, and aide time in minutes needed to accomplish a procedure. Total workload is determined by multiplying the work unit by the number of tests (raw count). (Karni et al.)

40. The major functions of a manager are

A. Planning, controlling, organizing, directing
B. Ordering supplies, directing, performance appraisal
C. Hiring, firing, performance appraisal, budget preparation
D. Budget preparation, directing, interfacing with physicians

The answer is A. A manager gets work done through others. To do this a manager must

1. Plan or determine goals and objectives
2. Organize the work required to fulfill the objectives
3. Direct or motivate employees to meet objectives
4. Control or measure performance and take corrective action

The four functions are performed simultaneously and continuously rather than as separate duties. (Karni et al.)

41. Effective delegation requires

A. Frequent reports in writing from the person carrying out delegated responsibilities
B. Close monitoring of the person to whom the responsibility is delegated
C. Delegation of enough authority to carry out responsibility
D. Delegation of minor responsibilities only

The answer is C. Delegation is the transfer of responsibility and authority to another person to accomplish tasks. Once a task has been delegated, the manager must allow the person to accomplish the objectives. (Karni et al.)

42. The evaluation of employee performance must relate back to

   A. A job description
   B. Verbal instructions
   C. The wage and salary program
   D. Recruitment practices

The answer is A. A job description clearly states what tasks an employee is to perform, specifies the manner in which they are to be carried out, and sets standards by which the adequacy of performance of each task can be assessed. (Karni et al.)

43. Statements of observable learning outcomes are called

   A. Goal statements
   B. Performance standards
   C. Objectives
   D. Test questions

The answer is C. Educational objectives are statements of learning outcomes stated in terms of observable learner behaviors. Statements of general purposes are termed goals. Achievement of objectives can be measured by construction of test questions that relate back to them. Objectives can be classified into three domains: cognitive, psychomotor, and affective. (McBride)

44. A test that is used to evaluate an individual's abilities against a predetermined standard is

   A. Norm-referenced
   B. Criterion-referenced
   C. Not valid
   D. Not reliable

The answer is B. A criterion-referenced test has a predetermined level set for passing. A norm-referenced test sets a passing score based on the performance of all the examinees taking the test at that time. A frequently calculated passing score for a norm-referenced examination is 1 SD below the mean. (McBride)

45. Which of the following statements concerning type I reagent grade water is true?

   A. It is not covered by NCCLS specifications for reagent grade water.
   B. It is recommended for use in procedures requiring minimal interference and maximal precision and accuracy.
   C. It may be used for washing glassware if followed by a rinse of higher reagent grade.
   D. It may be stored for extended periods of time after production without affecting its reagent grade.

The correct answer is B. The term *reagent grade water* is accompanied by a type I, II, or III designation. Type I has rigid specifications of purity established by the NCCLS and is recommended for those procedures requiring minimal interference and maximal precision and accuracy. These procedures include preparation of standards, as well as enzyme and electrolyte analyses. (Tietz, pp. 5–7)

46. Which of the following chemicals has been replaced in laboratory procedures because of its carcinogenic potential?

    A. Benzidine
    B. Xylene
    C. *o*-toluidine
    D. Methanol

The answer is A. Some chemicals that have been used freely in the laboratory are now known to be hazardous because they are carcinogenic. This includes benzidine, which was used for detecting the presence of hemoglobin. Benzidine can be replaced by other chemicals that are effective and much safer, such as tetramethylbenzidine. (Sonnenwirth et al.)

47. The amount of flammable and combustible liquids that may be stored in a laboratory is limited by

    A. Occupational Safety and Health Administration (OSHA) and National Fire Protection Association (NFPA) Standards
    B. The daily use of the laboratory
    C. The judgment of the supervisor
    D. Environmental Protection Agency (EPA) standards

The answer is A. Quantities are limited by OSHA and the NFPA. OSHA regulations limit the quantities allowed in any workplace, and NFPA standards further limit the quantities allowed in laboratories. The Joint Commission on Accreditation of Healthcare Organizations (JCAHO) and CAP have both adopted the NFPA standards. (Karni et al.)

48. An explosion-proof refrigerator

    A. Has a door that will withstand an explosion
    B. Has all electric switches outside the refrigeration compartment
    C. Operates at lower temperatures so vaporization does not occur
    D. Is vented so vapors will not collect in the refrigeration compartment

The answer is B. Explosion-proof refrigerators have all electric contacts on the outside of the refrigeration compartment. This is the only type of refrigerator suitable for the storage of flammable and combustible liquids. (Rose)

49. When there are five or six consecutive values that continue to increase or decrease on a Levey-Jennings chart, it is called a

A. Shift
B. Normal occurrence
C. Trend
D. Reliable measurement

The answer is C. A trend is a steadily increasing or decreasing control value. It occurs when the analytic method suffers a progressively developing problem. (Henry)

50. Which of the following may be included on an application form or in an interview without violating Equal Employment Opportunity Commission (EEOC) regulations?

A. Arrests
B. Marital status
C. Child care provisions
D. History of being disciplined or fired

The answer is D. Arrests are not convictions and no proof of a crime. It is not in violation to ask for convictions. Questions regarding marital status and child care provisions are in violation of the Equal Employment Opportunity Act of 1972. (Karni et al.)

References

Bauer, J.D. *Clinical Laboratory Methods* (9th ed.). St. Louis: Mosby, 1982.
Bruce, W.A. *Basic Quality Assurance and Quality Control in the Clinical Laboratory.* Boston: Little, Brown, 1984.
Campbell, J.B. *Laboratory Mathematics.* (3rd ed.). St. Louis: Mosby, 1984.
Handsfield, H. H. et. al., Prevalence of antibody to HIV and HBV in blood samples submitted to a hospital laboratory. *JAMA* 258:3395–3397, 1987.
Henry, H. B. (Ed.). *Clinical Diagnosis by Laboratory Methods* (17th ed.). Philadelphia: Saunders, 1984.
Karni, K. et. al. *Clinical Laboratory Management.* Boston: Little, Brown, 1982.
McBride, K. *Textbook of Clinical Laboratory Supervision.* New York: Appleton-Century-Crofts, 1982.
McNeely, M.D. *Microcomputer Applications in the Clinical Laboratory.* Chicago: ASCP Press, 1987.
Miller, B.M. *Laboratory Safety: Principles and Practices.* Washington, D.C.: American Society for Microbiology, 1986.
Rose, S.L. *Clinical Laboratory Safety.* Philadelphia: Lippincott, 1984.
Sonnenwirth, A.C., et. al. (Eds.). *Gradwohl's Clinical Laboratory Methods and Diagnosis* (8th ed.). St. Louis: Mosby, 1980.
Tietz, N.W. (Ed.). *Fundamentals of Clinical Chemistry* (3rd ed.).
Weisbrot, I.M. *Statistics for the Clinical Laboratory.* Philadelphia: Lippincott, 1985.

Review Tests 6

CLT Review Test

1. Which of these hormones lowers the blood glucose level?

    A. Cortisol
    B. Epinephrine
    C. Glucagon
    D. Insulin

(Tietz; Kaplan and Pesce; Bishop et al.).

2. If a lipemic serum is centrifuged and the creamy layer discarded before analysis, which of these errors will occur?

    A. The cholesterol result will be falsely high.
    B. The triglyceride result will be falsely low.
    C. Both the cholesterol and triglyceride results will be falsely high.
    D. Both the cholesterol and HDL cholesterol results will be falsely low.

(Tietz; Kaplan and Pesce; Bishop et al.)

3. A falsely elevated value for serum total protein is caused by

    A. Arterial blood
    B. Hemolysis
    C. Proteinuria
    D. A reclining patient

(Tietz; Bishop et al.)

4. An enzyme assay which shows substrate exhaustion should be repeated using

    A. Less sample
    B. Less substrate
    C. Longer light path
    D. Longer reaction time

(Tietz; Kaplan and Pesce; Bishop et al.)

5. The Jaffe reaction uses alkaline picrate to measure

    A. Ammonia
    B. Creatinine
    C. Urea
    D. Uric acid

(Tietz; Kaplan and Pesce; Bishop et al.)

6. Which vitamin is required for normal absorption of dietary calcium?

   A. Vitamin A
   B. Vitamin B_{12}
   C. Vitamin C
   D. Vitamin D

(Tietz; Kaplan and Pesce; Bishop et al.)

7. Which of these changes will occur if blood (from a patient who is breathing room air) is exposed to room air?

	pH	PCO_2	PO_2
A.	Increase	Decrease	Increase
B.	Increase	Increase	Decrease
C.	Decrease	Decrease	Increase
D.	Decrease	Increase	Decrease

(Tietz; Kaplan and Pesce; Bishop et al.)

8. Urine samples for quantitative measurement of trace metals should be collected

   A. After a 24-hr fast
   B. In an acid-rinsed container
   C. With boric acid added
   D. On ice to prevent degradation of urinary components

(Tietz; Kaplan and Pesce)

9. Decreased serum levels of total thyroxine (T_4), thyroid-stimulating hormone (TSH), and tri-iodothyronine resin uptake (T_3RU) indicate

   A. Euthyroidism with decreased thyroxine-binding globulin (TBG)
   B. Euthyroidism with excess TBG
   C. Primary hypothyroidism
   D. Secondary hypothyroidism

(Tietz; Kaplan and Pesce; Bishop et al.)

10. Which of these patterns of serum results is consistent with obstructive liver disease?

	Total bilirubin	Conjugated bilirubin	Total alkaline phosphatase
A.	↑	↑	↑
B.	↑	Normal	↑
C.	Normal	↑	↓
D.	↑	Normal	↓

(Tietz; Kaplan and Pesce; Bishop et al.)

11. The glucose level expected in normal spinal fluid is

   A. Less than 35 mg/dl
   B. 60 to 80% of the serum glucose level
   C. Equal to the serum glucose level
   D. Over 100 mg/dl

(Tietz; Bishop et al.)

12. The response of a PCO_2 electrode depends on

   A. Activity of bicarbonate ion
   B. Coulombs of current used
   C. Current flow in the presence of dissolved CO_2
   D. H^+ produced by CO_2 reacting with H_2O

(Tietz; Kaplan and Pesce; Bishop et al.)

13. The term *electroendosmosis*, as used in electrophoresis, describes

   A. An evaporation artifact
   B. Migration of buffer
   C. Production of heat
   D. Splitting of beta peak

(Tietz; Kaplan and Pesce; Bishop et al.)

14. Calculate the PCO_2 value that should be used for this calibrating gas:

   10.00 % CO_2
   Barometric pressure: 750 mm Hg
   Temperature: 37°C
   PH_2O: 47 mm Hg

   A. 70 mm Hg
   B. 75 mm Hg

C. 80 mm Hg
D. 100 mm Hg

(Tietz; Kaplan and Pesce)

15. Which one of these *is not* a colligative property of a solution?

A. Boiling temperature
B. Freezing temperature
C. Osmolality
D. pH

(Tietz; Kaplan and Pesce; Bishop et al.)

16. The proximal and distal convoluted tubules are separated anatomically by the

A. Bowman space
B. Collecting ducts
C. Juxtaglomerular apparatus
D. Loop of Henle

(Tietz; Kaplan and Pesce; Bishop et al.; Graff; Ross and Neely)

17. Serum urea concentration is increased by all *except*

A. Decreased renal blood flow
B. Diuresis
C. High protein diet
D. Renal failure

(Tietz; Kaplan and Pesce; Bishop et al.)

18. Which of these formed elements in urinary sediment indicates renal disease rather than lower urinary tract disease?

A. Granular casts
B. Erythrocytes
C. Leukocytes
D. Yeast

(Kaplan and Pesce; Graff; Ross and Neely)

19. The dipstick for urine specific gravity depends on the effect of

A. Binding of dye by buffer
B. Protein on the pK of the indicator
C. Ionic strength on the dissociation of the dye
D. The presence of ionic solutes

(Graff)

20. Which of these clearances is the most accurate measurement of glomerular filtration rate?

    A. Amylase clearance
    B. Creatinine clearance
    C. Phosphate clearance
    D. Urea clearance

(Tietz; Kaplan and Pesce; Bishop et al.)

21. Factors VII, IX, and X are not found in

    A. Whole blood
    B. Fresh citrated plasma
    C. Aged serum
    D. Barium sulfate–absorbed plasma

(Williams et al.)

22. Which of the following coagulation tests would *not* be included in a preoperative coagulation screening battery?

    A. Factor VIII assay
    B. Bleeding time
    C. Activated partial thromboplastin time (APTT)
    D. Prothrombin time (PT)

(Harker)

23. Most currently used automated coagulation instruments detect clot formation by a change in

    A. Optional density
    B. Ionic rate
    C. Electric conductivity
    D. Optical density or electric conductivity

(Lee)

24. A physician orders a factor IX assay. The screening test that has probably been performed and found to be abnormal is

    A. Bleeding time
    B. PT
    C. APTT
    D. Both PT and APTT

(Miale)

25. A normal APTT with a prolonged PT would indicate a possible deficiency in factor

A. II
B. X
C. VIII
D. VII

(Williams et al.)

26. Your last 20 Wright's-stained (Romanowsky) smears are all too pink in color. What is the best way to remedy this situation?

A. Make all blood smears thinner.
B. Increase the methanol content of the stain.
C. Shorten the staining (buffer) time.
D. Increase the pH of the buffer.

(Henry)

27. Red blood cells seen on a peripheral smear stained with Wright's stain contain inclusion bodies that are thought to be iron. What confirmatory stain should be done?

A. Brilliant cresyl blue
B. New methylene blue
C. Prussian blue
D. Feulgen

(Williams et al.)

28. Azurophilic granules first appear in which myelocytic stage?

A. Myeloblast
B. Promyelocyte
C. Myelocyte
D. Metamyelocyte

(Diggs et al.)

29. A supravital stain must be used to demonstrate the presence of

A. Howell-Jolly bodies
B. Siderocytes
C. Malarial parasites
D. Heinz bodies

(Brown)

30. An erroneously high hematocrit reading can be caused by

    A. Excessive centrifugation
    B. Hemolysis of the blood sample
    C. Reading the buffy coat as part of the packed cell portion
    D. Macrocytosis

(Henry)

31. The hematology supervisory technologist has asked you to recalibrate a standard curve for cyanmethemoglobin. The concentration of the standard solution is 60 mg/dl. The procedure requires that 0.02 ml blood be diluted in 5 ml reagent. If the undiluted standard is read directly as a calibration point, the equivalent hemoglobin concentration is

    A. 13.0 g/dl
    B. 14.0 g/dl
    C. 15.0 g/dl
    D. 16.0 g/dl

(Henry)

32. A patient has a chronic liver disease due to alcoholism. The MCV is normal, but on the peripheral blood smear many macrocytes are seen. What is the most likely explanation for this discrepancy?

    A. Many reticulocytes are present.
    B. The macrocytes seen are really codocytes.
    C. The cells are well filled with hemoglobin.
    D. The macrocytes are "thin" with an increase in diameter but normal cell volume.

(Wintrobe)

33. A patient's apparent packed cell volume (PCV) may be altered by all of the following *except*

    A. Speed of centrifugation
    B. Radius of centrifuge
    C. Length of time of centrifugation
    D. Amount of blood in the capillary tube

(Miale)

34. All dilution fluids for WBC counts must serve at least two purposes: One is to suspend and disperse the WBC. The other is to:

    A. Lyse RBCs
    B. Serve as a conductor for aperture current

C. Lyse platelets
D. Stain the nuclei

(Henry)

35. The ESR is affected by all of the following *except*

A. Fibrinogen level
B. Hematocrit
C. Type of hemoglobin
D. Anticoagulant-blood ratio

(Henry)

36. Heinz bodies would most likely be seen in a patient with

A. Iron deficiency anemia
B. Hereditary spherocytosis
C. Glucose-6-phosphate dehydrogenase deficiency
D. Megaloblastic anemia

(Wintrobe)

37. All of the following RBC morphology is assocated with splenectomy *except*

A. Nucleated red cells
B. Howell-Jolly bodies
C. Hypochromasia
D. Poikilocytosis

(Wintrobe)

38. Auer rods can be seen in all of the following leukemias *except*

A. Promyelocytic (M3)
B. Acute nonlymphoblastic (M1, M2)
C. Lymphoblastic (L1, L2, L3)
D. Monocytic (M4, M5)

(Williams et al.)

39. Which of the following statements is true concerning a normal WBC differential on an adult?

A. There are usually more lymphocytes than any other cell.
B. There are usually more monocytes than eosinophils.
C. There are usually more basophils than eosinophils.
D. There are usually more band neutrophils than lymphocytes.

(Henry)

40. The first step in performance of a spinal fluid cell count is to

    A. Dilute immediately.
    B. Plate directly onto the hematocytometer.
    C. Note color and clarity.
    D. Verify that the tube is the last one taken (tube 3).

(Henry)

41. The immunoglobulin class considered to be the most effective in fixing complement via the classic pathway is

    A. IgM
    B. IgA
    C. IgG
    D. IgE

(Stites et al.)

42. The cells in the immune system that are primarily involved in graft-versus-host reactions are

    A. B lymphocytes
    B. Macrophages
    C. Neutrophils
    D. T lymphocytes

43. The diagram below represents a typical immune response.

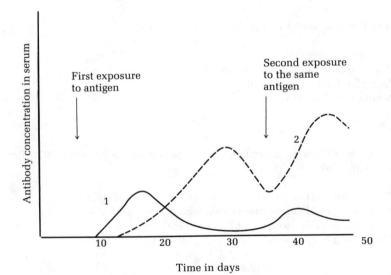

Time in days

Curve 1 indicates

A. Antibodies that do not directly agglutinate cells
B. A secondary response
C. IgM immunoglobulins
D. IgG immunoglobulins

(Bryant)

44. Treponemal tests such as the FTA-ABS test should be used

A. As screening tests for syphilis
B. For confirmatory testing for syphilis
C. To follow the efficacy of treatment
D. To test all blood donors for syphilis

(Rose et al.)

45. In a cold agglutinin titer, tube 1 contains 1.5 ml of saline and 0.5 ml of the patient's serum. Tubes 1 through 10 contain 1.0 ml of saline. The serum dilution in tube 1 is mixed and then 1.0 ml is transferred to tube 2. Twofold serial dilutions are continued through tube 9. What is the dilution of the patient's serum in tube 5?

A. 16
B. 32
C. 64
D. 128

(Bryant)

46. The neutralization test commonly used in the diagnosis of streptococcal infections detects which of the following substances in a patient's serum?

A. Antistreptolysin O
B. Streptolysin O
C. Streptolysin S
D. *Streptococcus pyrogenes*

(Bryant)

47. The most important mode of transmission of hepatitis B is

A. The parenteral (IV and mucosal) route
B. The fecal-oral route
C. Insect transmission
D. Transmission in contaminated water supplies

(Bryant)

48. Which of the following conditions may cause a false positive agglutination-inhibition test for pregnancy?

    A. Glycosuria
    B. Specific gravity of 1.005
    C. Proteinuria in excess of 1 g/24 hr
    D. Positive nitrite test

(Henry)

49. Heterophil antibodies that react with sheep erythrocytes after absorption with guinea pig kidney cells are found in infections with

    A. The Epstein-Barr virus
    B. The human immunodeficiency virus
    C. Cytomegalovirus
    D. *Listeria Monocytogenes*

(Bryant)

50. In an enzyme-linked immunoabsorbent assay (ELISA) the amount of bound antibody is quantitated by measuring the

    A. Optical density of the colored end product
    B. Amount of radioactivity
    C. Lysis of the indicator red cells
    D. Amount of fluorescence

(Roitt)

51. Which of the following persons would *not* qualify as a regular blood donor?

    A. Woman with a history of convulsions during a childhood illness that included a high fever
    B. Woman who is in the first trimester of pregnancy
    C. Man who had minor surgery 5 weeks ago
    D. Healthy man taking isoniazid because of a recent positive skin test for tuberculosis

(*Technical Manual of the American Association of Blood Banks*)

52. According to the American Association of Blood Banks (AABB) *Standards*, in addition to the full name and hospital number, a patient's blood sample for typing and compatibility testing must also be labeled with the

    A. Diagnosis
    B. Name of attending physician

C. Date of collection
D. Initials of the phlebotomist

(Standards for Blood Banks and Transfusion Services)

53. Serum for the majority of group A people contains

    A. Anti-A
    B. Anti-A,B
    C. Anti-B
    D. Anti-D

(Technical Manual of the American Association of Blood Banks)

54. The test used to detect in vivo coating of RBCs with immunoglobulin or complement is called the

    A. Direct antiglobulin test
    B. Hemagglutination inhibition test
    C. Indirect antiglobulin test
    D. Neutralization test

(Technical Manual of the American Association of Blood Banks)

55. A patient is group O, $Rh_o(D)$-positive. The patient's serum contains no unexpected antibodies. Which of the following donor units can be expected to be compatible in the crossmatch?

    A. A, $Rh_o(D)$-negative
    B. B, $Rh_o(D)$-negative
    C. O, $Rh_o(D)$-negative
    D. AB, $Rh_o(D)$-positive

(Technical Manual of the American Association of Blood Banks)

56. During interpretation of antibody cell panels, it is important to remember that M, N, and P_1 antibodies are most often identified

    A. At room temperature, 18°C, or 4°C
    B. By acidifying the serum
    C. After the antiglobulin test
    D. After enzymatic treatment of red cells

(Technical Manual of the American Association of Blood Banks)

57. Which of the following antigens gives enhanced reactions following treatment of red cells with proteolytic enzymes?

    A. Fy^a
    B. Rh$_o$
    C. N
    D. M

(Technical Manual of the American Association of Blood Banks)

58. The transfusion of which of the following blood components would be most effective in treating a patient with hemophilia who was experiencing a mild bleeding episode?

    A. Whole Blood
    B. Washed Red Blood Cells
    C. Platelet Concentrate
    D. Cryoprecipitate

(Technical Manual of the American Association of Blood Banks)

59. Given the following abbreviated cell panel, determine the most probable antibody or antibodies in the patient's serum.

	C	D	E	c	e	K	M	N	S	IS	37°C	AHG
1.	+	0	0	+	+	0	+	+	+	0	0	0
2.	+	+	0	0	+	0	+	0	+	0	0	0
3.	+	+	0	0	+	0	+	+	+	0	0	0
4.	0	+	+	+	0	+	+	0	+	0	0	1+
5.	0	0	+	+	+	0	+	+	0	0	0	0
6.	0	0	0	+	+	+	+	+	0	0	0	1+

Key: IS = initial spin; AHG = Antihuman globulin.)

    A. Anti-E
    B. Anti-c
    C. Anti-K
    D. Anti-E and anti-c

(Technical Manual of the American Association of Blood Banks)

60. If blood is required to prevent exsanguination (e.g., from a gunshot wound in an otherwise healthy man) and the blood type of the patient is not known, what is the product of choice?

    A. O-positive Packed Red Cells
    B. O-negative Packed Red Cells

C. O-positive Whole Blood
D. O-negative Whole Blood

(*Technical Manual of the American Association of Blood Banks*)

61. Gram-positive cocci in pairs and clusters are isolated from a superficial skin lesion. The isolate is beta-hemolytic on sheep blood agar. Further testing reveals that the isolate is catalase-positive and coagulase-positive. The definitive identification of this organism is

A. *Staphylococcus aureus*
B. *Staphylococcus epidermidis*
C. *Streptococcus agalactiae*
D. *Streptococcus pyogenes*

(Finegold et al.)

62. A transtracheal aspirate yields a pure culture of an alpha-hemolytic gram-positive coccus that is catalase-negative. The best test to perform in the subsequent identification process is

A. CAMP reaction
B. Coagulase
C. Susceptibility to bacitracin
D. Susceptibility to ethylhydrocupreine hydrochloride (optochin)

(Finegold et al.)

63. A child presents with a typical paroxysmal "whoop"-type cough and lymphocytosis. The most appropriate primary culture medium to isolate the suspected etiologic agent is

A. Charcoal yeast extract agar
B. Chocolate agar
C. Bordet-Gengou agar
D. Tinsdale agar

(Finegold et al.)

64. The organism that is the usual cause of severe obstructive epiglottitis, septicemia, and meningitis in young children is

A. *Haemophilus influenzae*
B. *Listeria monocytogenes*
C. *Neisseria meningitidis*
D. *Streptococcus pneumoniae*

(Lennette et al.)

65. Most members of the genus *Pseudomonas* are gram-negative rods that are

    A. Nonsaccharolytic and motile
    B. Motile and polar-flagellated
    C. Polar-flagellated and oxidase-negative
    D. Oxidase-positive and nonsaccharolytic

(Lennette et al.)

66. A microorganism resembling *Escherichia coli* is isolated from an infected traumatic wound. After additional tests the organism is identified as *Aeromonas hydrophila*. The single best test to differentiate *A. hydrophila* from *E. coli* is

    A. Gram stain
    B. Glucose fermentation
    C. Lactose fermentation
    D. Oxidase production

(Koneman et al.)

67. Which of the following species of *Mycobacterium* may be presumptively identified by demonstrating a positive niacin reaction?

    A. *Mycobacterium avium-intracellulare* complex
    B. *Mycobacterium bovis*
    C. *Mycobacterium tuberculosis*
    D. *Mycobacterium kansasii*

(Finegold et al.)

68. Which of the following specimens should not be routinely processed for anaerobic evaluation?

    A. Blood
    B. Clean, voided urine
    C. Synovial fluid
    D. Transtracheal aspirate

(Koneman et al.)

69. Chocolate agar is usually used as primary plating medium for

    A. Spinal fluid
    B. Adult throat
    C. Stool
    D. Urine

(Lennette et al.)

70. Several vacationers at a Gulf Coast seaside resort complain of severe abdominal pain and diarrhea after ingesting raw oysters. The agar that is most appropriate for screening these patients' stools is

A. Bismuth sulfite
B. Cellibiose arginine lysine
C. Cycloserine cefoxitin fructose
D. Thiosulfate citrate bile salts sucrose

(Lennette et al.)

71. The reagent(s) used to detect a positive indole reaction for the Entero-bacteriaceae is(are)

A. Alpha-naphthylamine and sulfanilic acid
B. Alpha-naphthol and potassium hydroxide
C. Paradimethylaminobenzaldehyde
D. Tetramethylparaphenylenediamine dihydrochloride

(Finegold et al.)

72. Which pair of organisms provides an appropriate quality control check for the biochemical reactions on eosin-methylene blue agar (EMB) and on Hektoen enteric (HE) agar?

A. *Escherichia coli, Klebsiella pneumoniae*
B. *Salmonella enteritidis, E. coli*
C. *Shigella sonnei, E. coli*
D. *Providencia rettgeri, K. pneumoniae*

(Finegold et al.)

73. A saprobic fungus whose micromorphology can be easily confused with that of *Histoplasma capsulatum* is

A. *Fusarium*
B. *Pseudoallescheria*
C. *Chrysosporium*
D. *Sepedonium*

(Koneman et al.)

74. A direct microscopic examination of an exudate from the lung reveals large spherules with endospores. The thick-walled spherules should alert the technologist to the possibility of

A. Cryptococcosis
B. Coccidioidomycosis
C. Candidiasis
D. Blastomycosis

(Lennette et al.)

75. A quality control regimen is to be selected for the following tests:

Phenylalanine deaminase (PAD)
Indole production
Voges-Proskauer (V-P)

Which pair of stock culture organisms would you select as suitable to verify the performance of these three tests?

A. *Klebsiella pneumoniae, Proteus vulgaris*
B. *P. vulgaris, Escherichia coli*
C. *E. coli, Enterobacter aerogenes*
D. *E. aerogenes, K. pneumoniae*

(Finegold et al.)

76. Which of the following parasites are most likely to be overlooked on a wet preparation and detected on a permanent stained slide?

A. Protozoa
B. Larvae
C. Helminth eggs
D. Proglottids

(Garcia et al., p. 19)

77. Several cysts and trophozoites are seen on trichrome stain permanent mount and on iodine preparation from stool concentrate. Which of the following are characteristic of *Entamoeba histolytica*?

A. Cysts with five to eight nuclei and chromatoid bodies with splintered ends
B. Trophozoites with one nucleus with an eccentric karyosome
C. Clean cytoplasm with the possibility of RBC inclusions
D. Granular vacuoles containing bacteria and debris

(Garcia et al.)

78. Which of the following organisms would most likely be seen in a urethral discharge?

A. *Balantidium coli*
B. *Enteromonas hominis*
C. *Giardia lamblia*
D. *Trichomonas vaginalis*

(Garcia et al.)

79. Which of the following situations would most likely produce falsely decreased zones of inhibition on a Kirby-Bauer disk-diffusion susceptibility
test?

   A. Use of an antimicrobial disk with a higher-than-recommended concen-
      tration of an antimicrobial
   B. Use of an inoculum that is too light
   C. Use of Mueller-Hinton agar thinner than 4 mm
   D. A 2-hr delay in placing antimicrobial disks on the seeded plate

(Lennette, et al.)

80. In a broth dilution test the lowest concentration of an antibiotic that produces an irreversible killing of the organism is called the minimal

   A. Antibiotic concentration
   B. Bactericidal concentration
   C. Inhibitory concentration
   D. Susceptible concentration

(Washington)

81. Which of the following formulas may be used to convert absorbance (Abs)
to percent transmittance (%T)?

   A. $Abs = 1 + \log \%T$
   B. $Abs = 2 - \log \%T$
   C. $\%T = \log T + \log A$
   D. $Abs = 1 - \log \%T$

(Henry)

82. The purpose of the didymium filter used with the broad-bandwidth spectrophotometer is to

   A. Align the galvanometer beam
   B. Produce monochromatic light
   C. Adjust the concentration range of the solution
   D. Check the wavelength calibration

(Tietz)

83. Beer's law states the absorbance of light is

   A. Directly proportional to the concentration of a substance
   B. Indirectly proportional to the concentration of a substance
   C. Directly proportional to the %T
   D. Directly proportional to the logarithm of the light transmitted

(Tietz)

84. A microscope has the following marks on the objective lens, $10 \times .25NA$, and a $10\times$ ocular. What is the total magnification?

    A. $100\times$
    B. $1,000\times$
    C. $25\times$
    D. $250\times$

(Sonnenwirth et al.)

85. A 0.5-ml aliquot of a 1:10 dilution of a substance is added to 9.5 ml of a diluent. What is the final dilution of the substance?

    A. 1:20
    B. 1:200
    C. 1:10
    D. 1:100

(Campbell)

86. When using an automatic pipet calibrated in the TC (to contain) mode

    A. It must be held horizontally when filling.
    B. Depress the piston to the first stop to fill and the second stop to empty.
    C. Depress the piston to the second stop to fill and the first stop to empty.
    D. Depress the piston to the second stop to both fill and empty.

(Sonnenwirth et al.)

87. The source of a class C fire is

    A. Electric
    B. Organic solvents
    C. Paper or trash
    D. Combustible metals

(Rose)

88. Which of the following terms identifies the chemical reagent with the highest purity?

    A. Analytic grade
    B. Purified
    C. Technical
    D. Laboratory grade

(Henry)

89. The following data are obtained from a spectrophotometric analysis that follows Beer's law up to 300 mg/dl:

Absorbance of standard = 0.250
Absorbance of unknown = 0.100
Concentration of standard = 100 mg/dl
Dilution of unknown = 1:10

What is the concentration of the unknown?

A. 250 mg/dl
B. 400 mg/dl
C. 2500 mg/dl
D. Cannot calculate because it exceeds the limits of Beer's law

(Campbell)

90. A stock standard of glucose contains 1 g/dl glucose in 0.25% benzoic acid. What dilution is necessary to prepare a working standard with a concentration of 100 mg/dl?

A. 1:10
B. 1:100
C. 1:500
D. 1:1000

(Campbell)

91. A stock glucose standard has a concentration of 10 mg/ml. Which of the following dilutions will yield a working standard of 100 mg/dl?

A. 0.01 ml of stock standard + 9.99 ml of benzoic acid
B. 0.1 ml of stock standard + 0.9 ml of benzoic acid
C. 0.1 ml of stock standard + 9.9 ml of benzoic acid
D. 0.2 ml of stock standard + 0.8 ml of benzoic acid

(Campbell)

92. A lipemic serum specimen gives an absorbance value of 0.520 for total protein measured by the biuret method. The lipemic serum specimen blank absorbance value is 0.060. The 5.9-g/dl protein standard has an absorbance value of 0.350. The total protein value of the serum specimen is

A. 7.8 g/dl
B. 6.8 g/dl
C. 6.5 g/dl
D. 5.6 g/dl

(Henry)

93. An analyte standard of 20 mg/ml has an absorbance of 0.200. What is the concentration of an unknown specimen diluted 1:10 that has an absorbance of 0.100?

    A. 40 g/dl
    B. 10 g/dl
    C. 40 mg/ml
    D. 10 mg/ml

(Henry)

94. Calculate the concentration in milliequivalents per liter for a solution of 80 mg/dl NaOH. (Atomic weights: Na = 23; O = 16; H = 1)

    A. 2 mEq/L
    B. 8 mEq/L
    C. 20 mEq/L
    D. 40 mEq/L

(Campbell)

95. A procedure calls for an incubation of 30°C. Your water bath has a thermometer that only reads in degrees Fahrenheit. What should the thermometer read when the water bath is at the correct temperature for this procedure?

    A. 22°F
    B. 36°F
    C. 62°F
    D. 86°F

(Campbell)

96. Which of the following conditions is most likely to be suitable for clearly observing a highly transparent specimen that has a refractive index near that of the surrounding medium?

    A. The condenser raised to the highest position, and the light lowered
    B. The condenser in the lowest position, and the light turned up
    C. The condenser in the highest position, and the light turned up
    D. The condenser in the lowest position, and the light turned down

(Sonnenwirth et al.)

97. The force required to separate two phases during centrifugation is identified as the:

   A. Relative centrifugal force (rcf)
   B. Revolutions per minute (rpm)
   C. Tachometer speed
   D. Relative electromagnetic speed (RES)

(Tietz)

98. When there are five or more consecutive values distributed on one side of the mean, it is known as a

   A. Shift
   B. Normal occurrence
   C. Trend
   D. Reliable measurement

(Henry)

99. When ordering reagents for quantitative chemical analysis, what grade of chemical should be purchased?

   A. Chemicaly pure
   B. Reagent grade
   C. USP grade
   D. Technical grade

(Henry)

100. A device using a light-sensitive layer which produces an electric current when light strikes it is a

   A. Meter
   B. Photocell
   C. Thermocouple
   D. Cathode lamp

(Tietz)

Key to CLT Review Test

1. D	26. D	51. B	76. A
2. B	27. C	52. C	77. C
3. B	28. B	53. C	78. D
4. A	29. D	54. A	79. D
5. B	30. C	55. C	80. B
6. D	31. C	56. A	81. B
7. A	32. D	57. B	82. D
8. B	33. D	58. D	83. A
9. D	34. A	59. C	84. A
10. A	35. C	60. D	85. B
11. B	36. C	61. A	86. B
12. D	37. C	62. D	87. A
13. B	38. C	63. C	88. A
14. A	39. B	64. A	89. B
15. D	40. D	65. B	90. A
16. D	41. A	66. D	91. B
17. B	42. D	67. C	92. A
18. A	43. C	68. B	93. B
19. C	44. B	69. A	94. C
20. B	45. C	70. D	95. D
21. D	46. A	71. C	96. D
22. A	47. A	72. B	97. A
23. D	48. C	73. D	98. A
24. C	49. A	74. B	99. B
25. D	50. A	75. A	100. B

CLS Review Test

1. Which of these conditions *is most likely* to be associated with hypoglycemia when untreated?

   A. Hyperplasia of the adrenal cortex
   B. Insulin-dependent diabetes mellitus
   C. Tumor of the pancreatic beta cells of the islets of Langerhans
   D. Malabsorbtion syndrome

(Tietz; Kaplan and Pesce; Bishop et al.)

2. A lipemic serum separates into a thick creamy layer above clear serum
after overnight refrigeration. Analysis gives these results (reference value
in parentheses):

   Triglyceride: 200 mg/dl (40–160)
   Cholesterol: 250 mg/dl (140–220)
   HDL cholesterol: 20 mg/dL (30–70)
   Lipoprotein electrophoresis shows markedly elevated chylomicrons

   Which of the following is an appropriate interpretation?

A. The cholesterol result should be much higher.
B. The HDL cholesterol result should be much higher.
C. The triglyceride result should be much higher.
D. The lipoprotein electrophoresis should show more abnormalities.

(Tietz; Kaplan and Pesce; Bishop et al.)

3. Chronic obstructive liver disease *is not* associated with an elevated serum level of

A. Albumin
B. Alkaline phosphatase
C. Conjugated bilirubin
D. Globulins

(Tietz; Kaplan and Pesce; Bishop et al.)

4. Which enzyme reaction can be measured spectrophotometrically at 340 nm using this indicator system?

ATP + glucose + hexokinase + NADP + G-6-PD→NADPH + other products

A. Amylase
B. Creatine kinase
C. Lactate dehydrogenase
D. Lipase

(Tietz; Kaplan and Pesce; Bishop et al.)

5. Creatinine can be measured by all *except*

A. Convert to creatine enzymatically; then use a reaction catalyzed by creatine kinase to measure the creatine.
B. Convert to urea with urease; then measure the urea.
C. Produce ammonia from creatinine enzymatically; then measure the ammonia.
D. React with alkaline picrate; then measure the orange chromogen.

(Tietz; Kaplan and Pesce; Bishop et al.)

6. Chronic gastric suction causes

A. Hyperkalemia
B. Hypochloremia
C. Hypoxia
D. Metabolic acidosis

(Tietz; Kaplan and Pesce; Bishop et al.)

7. The term *isohydric shift* describes

    A. Buffering of metabolic acid by hemoglobin
    B. Diffusion of bicarbonate and chloride ions across the RBC membrane
    C. Exchange of sodium and hydrogen ions across the renal tubular membrane
    D. Stimulation of oxygen release from oxyhemoglobin by 2,3-diphosphoglycerate

(Tietz; Kaplan and Pesce; Bishop et al.)

8. A blood ethanol result of 100 mg/dl indicates

    A. A value below the detection limits of the assay
    B. A probable false value if serum ketones are present
    C. Probable impairment of cognitive or motor skills
    D. A toxic level in most adults

(Tietz; Kaplan and Pesce; Bishop et al.)

9. Which of these patterns of results is consistent with primary hyperparathyroidism?

	Serum Ca	Serum P	Urine Ca	Urine P
A.	↑	↑	↑	↓
B.	↑	↓	↑	↑
C.	↓	↑	↓	↑
D.	↓	↓	↓	↓

(Tietz; Kaplan and Pesce; Bishop et al.)

10. The precursor of porphobilinogen is

    A. Delta-aminolevulinic acid
    B. Heme
    C. Porphyrin
    D. Urobilinogen

(Tietz; Kaplan and Pesce; Bishop et al.)

11. Electrophoretic separation of proteins in concentrated spinal fluid is often requested for the diagnosis of

    A. Bacterial meningitis
    B. Multiple myeloma
    C. Multiple sclerosis
    D. Intracerebral hemorrhage

(Tietz; Kaplan and Pesce; Bishop et al.)

12. Fluorometry uses all *except*

    A. Addition of internal standard
    B. Filter or monochromator to select the emitted wavelength
    C. Filter or monochromator to select the exciting wavelength
    D. Right angle in the light beam to avoid interference by transmitted light

(Tietz; Kaplan and Pesce; Bishop et al.)

13. If the amount of labeled ligand added to a competitive protein binding assay is accidently twice as much as the method calls for, the amount of

    A. Bound labeled ligand will decrease.
    B. Bound labeled ligand will increase.
    C. Free patient ligand will decrease.
    D. Free and bound labeled ligand will not be altered.

(Tietz; Kaplan and Pesce; Bishop et al.)

14. Calculate the percent carryover from these results

Cup No.	Sample	Result
1	100 standard	100
2	100 standard	101
3	100 standard	99
4	100 standard	100
5	20 standard	25
6	20 standard	20
7	20 standard	20
8	20 standard	20

    A. 1%
    B. 5%
    C. 20%
    D. 25%

(Kaplan and Pesce)

15. Which of these isotopes can be measured in a gamma scintillation counter?

    A. ^{14}C
    B. ^{3}H
    C. ^{125}I
    D. ^{16}O

(Tietz; Kaplan and Pesce)

16. Polyuria may be caused by

    A. Excess antidiuretic hormone secretion
    B. Hyperaldosteronism
    C. Narrowing of the renal artery
    D. Polydipsia

(Tietz, 690; Kaplan and Pesce; Bishop et al.)

17. Fat droplets may be seen in urinary sediment in all *except*

    A. Crush injuries involving subcutaneous fat
    B. Cystitis
    C. Major fractures of long bones
    D. Nephrotic syndrome

(Kaplan and Pesce; Graff)

18. The urine sample best suited for the dipstick nitrite test is

    A. Collected during the alkaline tide period
    B. Collected during painful urination
    C. Tested after 4 hr at room temperature
    D. The first morning sample

(Kaplan and Pesce; Graff; Ross and Neely)

19. The renal tissue that monitors renal blood supply and secretes renin is

    A. Bowman's capsule
    B. Glomerular tuft
    C. Juxtaglomerular apparatus
    D. Loop of Henle

(Tietz; Kaplan and Pesce; Bishop et al.; Ross and Neely)

20. The effect of aldosterone on renal tubules is to increase the

    A. Reabsorption of potassium
    B. Reabsorption of sodium
    C. Volume of glomerular filtrate
    D. Volume of urine per 24 hours

(Tietz; Kaplan and Pesce; Bishop et al.; Graff; Ross and Neely)

21. Protamine sulfate neutralizes which of the following anticoagulants?

    A. Coumarin
    B. EDTA

C. Sodium citrate
D. Heparin

(Harker)

22. Which clinical symptom is most frequently associated with thrombocytopenia?

   A. Thrombosis
   B. Hemarthroses
   C. Petechiae
   D. Deep hematomas

(Henry)

23. The APTT is usually prolonged in all of the following *except*

   A. Factor VIII deficiency
   B. Vitamin K deficiency
   C. Idiopathic thrombocytopenia
   D. Heparin therapy

(Henry)

24. A patient has a normal PT, and an abnormal APTT that is not corrected by either factor VIII-deficient or factor IX-deficient plasma. The best explanation for this situation would be

   A. Factor XI or XII deficiency
   B. Fibrinogen deficiency
   C. Technical error
   D. A circulating antibody to factor VIII

(Miale)

25. In which of the activation steps of current coagulation theory does phospholipid play a role?

   A. X→Xa
   B. IX→IXa
   C. Fibrinogen to fibrin
   D. XII→XIIa

(Henry)

26. A patient has been in the hospital for 10 days receiving IV fluid replacement and being treated with antibiotics for pneumonia. The coagulation results include a prolonged PT, prolonged APTT, normal thrombin time, normal platelet count, and normal factor V level. The most probable diagnosis of this patient is

    A. Liver disease
    B. Disseminated intravascular coagulation
    C. Vitamin K deficiency
    D. Afibrinogenemia

(Wintrobe)

27. Red blood cells seen on a peripheral smear stained with Wright's stain contain inclusion bodies that are thought to be iron. Which confirmatory stain should be done?

    A. Brilliant cresyl blue
    B. New methylene blue
    C. Prussian blue
    D. Feulgen

(Williams et al.)

28. A patient has a WBC count of 80×10^9/L. The peripheral blood smear shows 90% blasts, 8% lymphocytes, and 2% neutrophils. Cytochemical stains requested by the hematologist revealed the following:

PAS: negative
Sudan B: 85% positive
Alpha-naphthyl acetate: positive
Naphthol AS-D chloroacetate: positive
Naphthol AS-D acetate: positive
Naphthol AS-D acetate with NaF: negative

What is the most likely diagnosis?

    A. Acute lymphoblastic leukemia
    B. Acute monoblastic leukemia
    C. Acute myeloblastic leukemia
    D. Erythroleukemia

(Henry)

29. One of the characteristic findings for the diagnosis of chronic myelogenous leukemia is

    A. A positive nitroblue tetrazolium test
    B. An elevated leukocyte alkaline phosphatase score
    C. The Philadelphia chromosome
    D. A positive tartrate-resistant acid phosphatase reaction

(Williams et al.)

30. All of the following are associated with anemia of chronic disorders *except*

    A. Hypochromic, microcytic erythrocytes
    B. Adequate iron stores
    C. Reduced concentration of transferrin
    D. Normal serum iron

(Williams et al.)

31. Which of the following is *not* found in hereditary spherocytosis?

    A. Extravascular hemolysis
    B. Increased osmotic fragility
    C. Positive Coombs' test
    D. Usually, an MCHC greater than 35 g/100 ml

(Williams et al.)

32. All of the following statements are true of the fibrinolytic system *except*

    A. Plasmin functions to keep the vascular system free of deposited fibrin or fibrin clots.
    B. The active enzyme of the system is plasmin.
    C. Plasmin is not normally found circulating in plasma.
    D. Fibrinolysis is decreased whenever coagulation is increased.

(Henry)

33. A child has ingested rat poison. Which of the following tests should be performed to assess the effect of the poison on the patient's coagulation mechanism?

    A. Prothrombin time (PT)
    B. Fibrin degradation products (FDP)
    C. Fibrinogen
    D. Platelet count

(Henry)

34. With which disease do the following erythrocyte indices correlate best?

MCV: 126 fl
MCH: 42 pg
MCHC: 33 g/dl

A. Iron deficiency anemia
B. Rheumatoid arthritis
C. Sickle cell anemia
D. Folate deficiency

(Wintrobe)

35. A man has an RBC count of $4.00 \times 10^{12}/L$ and an absolute reticulocyte count of $7.40 \times 10^9/L$. These may be indicative of

A. Iron deficiency
B. Hemolytic disease
C. Inadequate marrow stimulation
D. Normality

(Henry)

36. A patient is admitted to the emergency room with extensive burns. Expected erythrocyte morphologic features would include

A. Microspherocytes
B. Acanthocytes
C. Hypochromasia
D. Codocytes (target cells)

(Wintrobe)

37. The following results were obtained on a leukocyte alkaline phosphatase stain:

No. of cells	Score
3	0
20	1
41	2
24	3
12	4

These results would indicate

A. Myelogenous leukemia
B. Lymphocytic leukemia

C. Paroxysmal nocturnal hemoglobinuria
D. Leukemoid reaction

(Miale)

38. Examination of a Wright's-stained bone marrow smear reveals many large cells (20–80 μm) with globular cytoplasmic inclusions. Cytochemical analysis of the cell content confirms the presence of ceroid, cholesterol, and sphingomyelin. The cells are most likely

   A. Diagnostic of Niemann-Pick disease
   B. Positive on peroxidase staining
   C. Diagnostic of Alder's anomaly
   D. Diagnostic of Chédiak-Higashi syndrome

(Miale)

39. A long bleeding time, low factor VIII activity, reduced platelet aggregation with ristocetin, and low platelet adhesiveness are characteristic of:

   A. Classic hemophilia (A)
   B. Christmas disease
   C. von Willebrand's disease
   D. Disseminated intravascular coagulation

(Miale)

40. Which of the following radioactive substances is correctly matched with the test in which it is used?

   A. ^{12}B: Schilling test
   B. ^{51}Cr: kinetic iron studies
   C. ^{12}B: red cell survival studies
   D. ^{57}Fe: blood volume

(Henry)

41. According to Coombs and Gell, the hypersensitivity reaction characterized by the release of pharmacologic mediators such as histamine by IgE-sensitized mast cells is classified as

   A. Type I
   B. Type II
   C. Type III
   D. Type IV

(Roitt)

42. In the alternate complement pathway, the first component to be activated is

    A. C1
    B. C2
    C. C3
    D. C4

(Roitt)

43. The following figure represents a radial immunodiffusion plate for quanti-
    tating IgG.

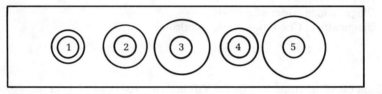

    Wells 1 to 3 contain reference standards, each equal to the following:

    1. 700 mg%
    2. 1,400 mg%
    3. 2,800 mg%

    The other wells contain unknowns. What can be said about precipitin ring
    5?

    A. It should be measured and plotted on the standard line by extending the
       line beyond 2,800.
    B. It probably represents a situation in which extra sample was spilled on
       the surface of the gel, but it still can be measured.
    C. It represents a patient sample that is too high and must be diluted (e.g.,
       1:2) and run again.
    D. It represents a ring typically seen from a patient with
       agammaglobulinemia.

(Stites et al.)

44. A blood sample for a cold agglutinin titer is stored at 4°C overnight and
    tested in the morning. The results of this cold agglutinin titer will be

    A. Falsely lowered due to the 4°C incubation
    B. Unaffected by incubation at 4°C
    C. Falsely elevated due to enhancement of cold antibodies
    D. Falsely elevated due to complement activation

(Bryant)

45. Nontreponemal tests for syphilis have a high incidence of biologic false positive results. Which of the following disorders frequently result(s) in a biologic false positive VDRL test?

A. Hypogammaglobulinemia
B. Iron deficiency anemia
C. Systemic lupus erythematosus
D. Hemophilia A

(Henry)

46. A patient's serum is absorbed with guinea pig kidney and beef RBCs and then titered with sheep RBCs in the heterophil absorption test. Absorption with guinea pig kidney has no effect on the sheep RBC titer, but beef RBC absorption causes a fourfold drop in antisheep RBC titer. This situation indicates

A. Laboratory error
B. Serum sickness
C. A noninfectious mononucleosis viral disease
D. Infectious mononucleosis

(Stites et al.)

47. In an antistreptolysin O test, the hemolysin (streptolysin) control tube shows partial lysis. How would this most likely affect the results of the antistreptolysin O test?

A. By causing falsely high values due to decreased hemolysis
B. By causing falsely low values due to increased hemolysis
C. No effect, since the hemolysis would be distributed equally among all tubes
D. No effect, since the test is read as the lack of hemolysis

(Rose et al.)

48. A positive test for antibodies directed against cell nuclei (ANA) is associated with a diagnosis of

A. Autoimmune hemolytic anemia
B. Hashimoto's disease
C. Pernicious anemia
D. Systemic lupus erythematosus

(Bryant)

49. The HLA-DR antigens are detected using which of the following procedures?

   A. One-way mixed lymphocyte cultures
   B. Microcytotoxicity assays with purified B lymphocytes
   C. Primed lymphocyte tests
   D. Complement fixation assays using T cell–enriched populations

(Stites et al.)

50. Confirmatory testing for the antibody to the human immunodeficiency virus (HIV) is performed using which of the following procedures?

   A. ELISA
   B. Indirect immunofluorescence
   C. Radioimmunoassay
   D. Western blot techniques

(Rose et al.)

51. Exceptions to regular blood donation requirements can be made for

   A. Paid donors
   B. Pregnant women
   C. Healthy athletes
   D. Donations for autologous transfusion

(Technical Manual of the American Association of Blood Banks)

52. The following reactions are obtained on ABO testing of a patient's blood sample. What is the most likely ABO group?

Reagent	Anti-A	Anti-B	Anti-A$_1$ lectin	A$_1$ cells	A$_2$ cells	B cells	O cells
Patient	3+	negative	negative	2+	negative	4+	negative

   A. A$_1$
   B. A$_3$
   C. A$_2$ with anti-A$_1$
   D. A$_2$B with anti-A$_1$

(Technical Manual of the American Association of Blood Banks)

53. A patient's red cells type as group O, but the serum types as group A. Secretor tests are performed on the saliva with the following results:

   (Anti-A + saliva) + A$_1$ cells: O
   (Anti-B + saliva) + B cells: 3+
   (Anti-H + saliva) + O cells: + w

Choose the correct ABO type for this patient.

A. A (subgroup)
B. B
C. O
D. Cannot be determined

(Technical Manual of the American Association of Blood Banks)

54. When transfused, a person of phenotype rr will *not* produce the antibody

A. Anti-C
B. Anti-D
C. Anti-E
D. Anti-c

(Technical Manual of the American Association of Blood Banks)

55. The antibody least likely to show dosage is

A. Anti-D
B. Anti-M
C. Anti-Fy^a
D. Anti-Jk^a

(Technical Manual of the American Association of Blood Banks)

56. A 44-year-old man needs 3 units of blood for back surgery. The patient's cells fail to react with anti-A and anti-B; his serum reacts with A, B, and O cells. What is the next logical step to resolve this problem?

A. Identify the antibody or antibodies using a panel of O cells.
B. Perform an autoabsorption using the patient's own cells.
C. Titer the serum against the autologous control as well as random donor units. Compare the results and choose the least incompatible units.
D. Crossmatch the patient's serum with random donor cells at 37°C.

(Technical Manual of the American Association of Blood Banks)

57. A 23-year-old woman is found to have a positive antibody screen during a prenatal workup. Which of the following techniques would be most useful in determining if the antibody involved could cause hemolytic disease of the newborn?

A. Treating the maternal serum with 2-mercaptoethanol
B. The one-stage papain procedure
C. The two-stage papain procedure
D. The absorption-elution technique

(Technical Manual of the American Association of Blood Banks)

58. Which of the following must be done immediately to investigate a possible hemolytic transfusion reaction?

    A. Determine patient ABO and Rh types of prereaction and postreaction specimens.
    B. Examine a postreaction urine specimen for free hemoglobin.
    C. Perform an antibody screening test and crossmatch using the prereaction specimen, the postreaction specimen, and the donor unit.
    D. Inspect the blood bank records and the label on the donor unit for possible clerical errors.

(*Technical Manual of the American Association of Blood Banks*)

59. Which of the following sets of reactions would be most consistent with the presence of anti-I? (Testing is carried out at 4°C.)

	Patient serum + patient cells	Patient serum + normal adult cells	Patient serum + cells from cord blood
A.	4+	4+	0
B.	4+	4+	4+
C.	1+	4+	4+
D.	1+	2+	1+

(*Technical Manual of the American Association of Blood Banks*)

60. A request for 3 units of packed cells is made for a male patient, aged 80 years, for surgery to repair a broken hip. He is typed as O, Rh_o-negative. His antibody screening test shows a reaction in the antiglobulin (AHG) phase. A transfusion history indicates he received 2 units of whole blood in 1979. The results of the antibody panel are shown below.

	C	D	E	c	e	K	k	Fy^a	Fy^b	Jk^a	Jk^b	M	N	S	Test Results AHG
1	+	0	0	+	+	0	+	0	+	+	0	+	+	+	1+
2	+	+	0	0	+	0	+	+	+	+	0	+	0	+	1+
3	+	+	0	0	+	0	+	0	+	0	+	+	+	+	0
4	0	+	+	+	0	+	+	0	+	+	+	+	0	+	1+
5	0	0	+	+	+	0	+	+	+	+	+	+	+	0	1+
6	0	0	0	+	+	+	0	+	0	0	+	0	+	0	0

The antibody in this patient's serum is most likely

    A. Anti-C
    B. Anti-D
    C. Anti-Jk^a
    D. Anti-Jk^b

(*Technical Manual of the American Association of Blood Banks*)

61. An isolate from a urinary tract infection grows as a porcelain-white, butyrous colony that is nonhemolytic on sheep blood agar. The isolate is a catalase-positive, gram-positive coccus. Biochemical testing reveals the following reactions:

Tube coagulase: negative   Mannitol: acid
Acid from anaerobic glucose: weak   Trehalose: acid
Novobiocin sensitivity: resistant

This isolate is best

A. Identified as a *Micrococcus* species
B. Identified as *Staphylococcus epidermidis*
C. Identified as *Staphylococcus saprophyticus*
D. Reworked to resolve the discrepancy

(Lennette et al.)

62. A sputum culture yields predominantly alpha-hemolytic, flat colonies on sheep blood agar that on Gram stain reveal gram-positive cocci in pairs. Which biochemical tests will aid in the identification of this isolate?

A. Bacitracin and sulfamethoxazole-trimethoprim susceptibility
B. Bile esculin hydrolysis and 6.5% NaCl tolerance
C. Catalase test and CAMP reaction
D. Optochin susceptibility or bile solubility

(Finegold et al.)

63. A catalase-negative non-hemolytic gram-positive coccus isolated from a urine specimen from a 42-year-old woman hydrolyzes bile esculin and grows in the presence of 6.5% NaCl. This isolate could be the species

A. *Streptococcus durans*
B. *Streptococcus faecalis*
C. *Streptococcus pneumoniae*
D. Alpha-hemolytic streptococcus viridans group

(Finegold et al.)

64. To establish a definitive diagnosis of diphtheria, which of the following must be confirmed?

A. Biochemical test results
B. Methylene blue micromorphology
C. Tellurite reduction
D. Toxin production

(Finegold et al.)

65. The following results are obtained from a nonlactose-fermenting, gram-negative rod isolated from a urinary tract infection:

Triple sugar iron: alk/acid   Citrate: negative
H_2S: negative   Phenylalanine deaminase: positive
Indole: positive   Urease: positive
Motility: positive   Ornithine: positive

The identity of this organism is

A. *Morganella morganii*
B. *Proteus mirabilis*
C. *Providencia alcalifaciens*
D. *Providencia stuartii*

(Finegold et al.)

66. A green colony type with black center on Hektoen agar is inoculated to a stool screen using triple sugar iron (TSI) agar, lysine iron agar (LIA), and Christensen's urease. The following reactions develop:

TSI: alkaline/acid and gas, H_2S-positive
LIA: lysine-positive, H_2S-positive
Urease: negative

These results are consistent with a species of

A. *Citrobacter*
B. *Escherichia*
C. *Proteus*
D. *Salmonella*

(Finegold et al.)

67. A patient diagnosed as having nonspecific vaginitis complains of malodorous vaginal discharge. A direct smear of the vaginal exudate on Gram stain reveals epithelial cells that are covered with masses of small gram-variable coccobacillary rods suggestive of "clue" cells. This finding is indicative of

A. *Chlamydia trachomatis*
B. *Gardnerella vaginalis*
C. *Neisseria gonorrhoeae*
D. *Lactobacillus* species

(Lennette et al.)

68. In the diagnosis of primary atypical pneumonia, it must be established of the suspected causative agent that

A. Subcultures grow on serum-free media.
B. The organism grows on sheep blood agar.

C. The colony stains acid-fast.

D. The agent is a *Mycoplasma*.

(Lennette et al.)

69. From a sputum specimen, an acid-fast bacillus grows on Löwenstein-Jensen medium for 18 days at 35°C capneic incubation. Initially, the colonies are buff, raised, and rough when grown in the dark. After exposure to light, no change in pigmentation is detectable. On examination under 10x magnification and on stain, serpentine cording is seen. Which of the following characteristics confirm the identity of the most likely etiologic agent?

A. Niacin-positive, nitrate-positive

B. Niacin-negative, nitrate-positive

C. Niacin-positive, nitrate-negative

D. Niacin-negative, nitrate-negative

(Lennette et al.)

70. A gram-negative rod is inoculated into nitrate broth and incubated for 24 hr. After equal amounts of alpha-naphthylamine and sulfanilic acid are added, no color develops. Zinc dust is added and still no color develops. What action should you take?

A. Make up new reagents and check with quality control stains.

B. Repeat the nitrate test after 48 hr of incubation.

C. Interpret the results as negative.

D. Interpret the results as positive.

(Lennette et al.)

71. Sodium polyanetholsulfonate is added to blood culture media to

A. Prevent clotting

B. Activate complement activity

C. Enhance phagocytosis

D. Enhance the growth of fastidious pathogens

(Lennette et al.)

72. Which of the following bacterial species is unacceptable for performing quality control testing of anaerobic jars or glove boxes?

A. *Bacteroides melaninogenicus*

B. *Clostridium novyi*

C. *Clostridium tertium*

D. *Peptostreptococcus anaerobius*

(Lennette et al.)

73. *Blastomyces dermatitidis* can be differentiated from the saprobic species of *Chrysosporium* and *Pseudoallescheria* by

    A. Rapid growth of the colony
    B. Single conidia produced directly from hyphae or conidiophores
    C. Ability to convert to a yeast phase at 37°C
    D. Inability to grow on media containing cycloheximide and chloramphenicol

(Koneman et al.)

74. Persistent athlete's foot plagues a local baseball team in training season. A study is undertaken to identify the organism from each team member with typical signs of the fungal disease. The organism grows out in 12 days on Sabouraud's dextrose agar and Sabouraud's with chloramphenicol and cycloheximide as a snowy-white velvety colony with an undistinguished reverse. Rare long, narrow, smooth-walled macroconidia are seen on microscopic preparation. Thin, clavate, teardrop-shaped microconidia are borne laterally. Based on these data, a likely etiologic agent is

    A. *Microsporum audouinii*
    B. *Microsporum canis*
    C. *Trichophyton mentagrophytes*
    D. *Trichophyton rubrum*

(Koneman et al.)

75. The purpose of the iodine solution used in the direct preparation technique for screening stool specimens is to

    A. Enhance morphologic detail of organisms
    B. Check for motility of trophozoites
    C. Precipitate fecal material
    D. Stain debris, rather than parasites

(Garcia et al.)

76. An important cause of pneumonia in patients with acquired and congenital immunologic disorders and seen most recently in the male homosexual population is the organism that in a lung impression smear stained with Giemsa stain reveals eight nuclei scattered in a rosette formation. The identity of this organism is

    A. *Toxoplasma gondii*
    B. *Pneumocystis carinii*
    C. *Babesia*
    D. *Sarcocystis*

(Lennette et al.)

77. *Babesia* may infect humans and multiply in red cells; however, it can be differentiated from malarial agents because *Babesia*

   A. Has crescent-shaped gametocytes
   B. Forms hemozoin pigment in red cells
   C. Also occurs in leukocytes
   D. Develops ring forms and maltese cross forms

(Koneman)

78. A patient with a mild pneumonia that is suggestive of ornithosis would be infected with

   A. *Chlamydia psittaci*
   B. *Chlamydia trachomatis*
   C. *Mycoplasma pneumoniae*
   D. Rhinovirus

(Lennette et al.)

79. Cell culture media have antibiotics as ingredients to

   A. Enhance cell penetration
   B. Sterilize the medium
   C. Increase the cytopathic effect
   D. Reduce bacterial contamination

(Fenner and White)

80. To develop a minimum inhibitory concentration (MIC) procedure by macro-broth tube dilution you need to determine the required concentration of antimicrobial for preparation of working stock solution. The highest concentration of antimicrobial to be tested will be 128 μg/ml. Two milliliters of stock are transferred directly to the first tube and twofold serial dilutions are prepared in subsequent tubes. One milliliter of standardized inoculum is added to each tube. Based on these parameters, the concentration of antimicrobial in the working stock solution must be

   A. 256 μg/ml
   B. 512 μg/ml
   C. 1024 μg/ml
   D. Cannot be calculated from these data

(Lennette et al.)

81. According to organizational theorists, the functions of management include all of the following *except*

   A. Planning
   B. Motivating
   C. Organizing
   D. Purchasing

(Karni et al.)

82. Which of the following guarantees hospital employees the right to engage in collective bargaining?

   A. Wagner Act
   B. Clinical Laboratory Improvement Act (CLIA)
   C. National Labor Relations Act
   D. Taft-Hartley Act

(Karni et al.)

83. An employee performance evaluation accomplishes all of the following *except*

   A. Help determine training needs
   B. Help improve overall performance
   C. Allow an effective way to reprimand a problem employee
   D. Give an employee feedback on accomplishment of performance standards

(Karni et al.)

84. Dark-field microscopy is accomplished by

   A. Decreasing the intensity of the light source
   B. Lowering the condenser
   C. Closing the aperture on the condenser
   D. Using a light ring in the condenser to supply oblique light

(Sonnenwirth et al.)

85. Mainframe laboratory computers are usually connected to terminals via a

   A. Serial interface
   B. Parallel interface
   C. Data bus
   D. Modem

(McNeely)

86. Which of the following is used to measure the rpm of a centrifuge?

   A. Ohmmeter
   B. Rheostat
   C. Voltmeter
   D. Tachometer

(Henry)

87. The statistical test used to determine if two means are significantly different from one another is the

    A t test
    B. Standard deviation
    C. Coefficient of variation
    D. Correlation coefficient

(Henry)

88. A potentiometer is the same as a

    A. Variable resistor
    B. Capacitor
    C. Transformer
    D. Phototube

(Sonnenwirth et al.)

89. The percentage of normally distributed population that is expected to fall *outside* of 2 SDs is

    A. 2.5%
    B. 5%
    C. 15%
    D. 95%

(Campbell)

90. The danger of explosion from highly flammable solvents may be reduced by all of the following *except*

    A. Disposal of flammable solvents in the sewer with large quantities of water
    B. Using a fume hood
    C. Storing at temperatures below their flashpoint
    D. Maintaining small quantities outside of a flammable storage cabinet

(Tietz)

91. The coefficient of variation is

    A. Equal to the variance
    B. Expressed in the same units as the constituent being measured
    C. The ratio of the standard deviation to the mean value
    D. The scatter of values about the mean

(Henry)

92. Under a normal distribution curve, 68% of all results would represent how many standard deviations?

    A. 1
    B. 2
    C. 3
    D. 4

(Henry)

93. From these data what can be concluded about methods A and B?

Method	Mean (mg/dl)	SD (mg/dl)
A	102	5
B	42	2

    A. Method B is more precise than method A.
    B. Method A has more relative variability than method B.
    C. Method B is more accurate than method A.
    D. There is no significant difference in the relative variability of the methods.

(Weisbrot)

94. The degree of precision of a measurement determined from statistical considerations of the distribution of random error is best expressed in terms of

    A. Weighted average
    B. t test
    C. Standard deviation
    D. Linear regression

(Henry)

95. The sensitivity of a test method is determined by the

    A. Percentage of positive tests in patients known to have the disease
    B. Percentage of negative tests in people known not to have the disease
    C. Number of positive tests when the substance being measured is present in low concentration
    D. Number of true positives divided by the number of true negatives

(Henry)

96. Scores on the NCA examination are

   A. Set at 1 SD below the mean
   B. Based on the performance of all examinees taking the test at that time
   C. Based on a predetermined passing level
   D. Norm-referenced

(Karni et al.)

97. Careful examination of workload tallies does *not* assist in assessing

   A. Productivity
   B. Staffing needs
   C. Instrument downtime
   D. Time needed for each test

(Karni et al.)

98. Which of the following may be legally included on an employment application?

   A. Request for a photograph
   B. Credit rating
   C. Arrest record
   D. History of being disciplined or fired

(Karni et al.)

99. A series of measurements are 3, 8, 5, 1, 3, 11, and 4. What is the mean?

   A. 7
   B. 4
   C. 5
   D. 3

(Campbell)

100. A measurement, taken at an angle to the incident beam, of the amount of light scattered or reflected by small particles in a sample cuvette is the principle of

   A. Fluorometry
   B. Nephelometry
   C. Turbidimetry
   D. Mass spectrophotometry

(Tietz)

Key to CLS Review Test

1. C	26. C	51. D	76. B
2. C	27. C	52. C	77. D
3. A	28. B	53. A	78. A
4. B	29. C	54. D	79. D
5. B	30. D	55. A	80. A
6. B	31. C	56. A	81. D
7. A	32. D	57. A	82. C
8. C	33. A	58. D	83. C
9. B	34. D	59. A	84. D
10. A	35. B	60. C	85. A
11. C	36. A	61. C	86. D
12. A	37. D	62. D	87. A
13. B	38. A	63. B	88. A
14. D	39. C	64. D	89. B
15. C	40. A	65. A	90. A
16. D	41. A	66. D	91. C
17. B	42. C	67. B	92. A
18. D	43. C	68. D	93. D
19. C	44. A	69. A	94. C
20. B	45. C	70. D	95. A
21. D	46. D	71. A	96. C
22. C	47. A	72. C	97. C
23. C	48. D	73. C	98. D
24. D	49. B	74. D	99. C
25. A	50. D	75. A	100. B

References

Bishop, M.L., Duben-Von Laufen, J.L., and Fody, E.P. (Eds.), *Clinical Chemistry Principles, Procedures, Correlations.* Philadelphia: Lippincott, 1985.

Brown, B.A. *Hematology: Principles and Procedures* (5th ed.). Philadelphia: Lea & Febiger, 1988.

Bryant, N.J. *Laboratory Immunology and Serology* (2nd ed.). Philadelphia: Saunders, 1986.

Campbell, J.B. *Laboratory Mathematics* (3rd ed.). St. Louis: Mosby, 1984.

Diggs, L.W., et al. *The Morphology of Human Blood Cells* (3rd ed.). Chicago: Abbott Laboratories, 1985.

Fenner, F.J. and White, D.O. *Medical Virology* (2nd ed.). New York: Academic Press, 1976.

Finegold, S.M., et al. *Bailey and Scott's Diagnostic Microbiology* (7th ed.). St. Louis: Mosby, 1986.

Garcia, L.S., et al. *Diagnostic Parasitology: Clinical Laboratory Manual* (2nd ed.). St. Louis: Mosby, 1979.

Graff, L. *A Handbook of Routine Urinalysis,* Philadelphia, Lippincott, 1983.

Harker, L. *Hemostasis Manual* (3rd ed.). Philadelphia: Davis, 1983.

Henry, J.B. (Ed.). *Clinical Diagnosis and Management by Laboratory Methods* (17th ed.). Philadelphia: Saunders, 1984.

Koneman, E.W., et al. *Color Atlas and Textbook of Diagnostic Microbiology* (3rd ed.). Philadelphia: Lippincott, 1988.

Karni, K., et al. *Clinical Laboratory Management.* Boston: Little, Brown, 1982.

Lee, L.W. *Elementary Principles of Laboratory Instruments* (5th ed.). St. Louis: Mosby, 1983.

Lennette, E.H., et al. *Manual of Clinical Microbiology* (4th ed.). Washington, D.C.: American Society for Microbiology, 1985.

McNeely, M.D. *Microcomputer Applications in the Clinical Laboratory*. Chicago: ASCP Press, 1987.

Miale, J.B. *Laboratory Medicine: Hematology* (2nd ed.). Philadelphia: Lippincott, 1979.

Roitt, I. *Essential Immunology* (6th ed.). Oxford: Blackwell, 1988.

Rose, N.R., Friedman, H., and Fahey, J.L. (Eds.). *Manual of Clinical Immunology* (3rd ed.). Washington, D.C.: American Society for Microbiology, 1986.

Rose, S.L. *Clinical Laboratory Safety*. Philadelphia: Lippincott, 1984.

Ross, D.L., and Neely, A.E. *Textbook of Urinalysis and Body Fluids*. Norwalk, Conn.: Appleton-Century-Crofts, 1983.

Sonnenwirth, A.C., et al. (Eds.). *Gradwohl's Clinical Laboratory Methods and Diagnosis* (8th ed.). St. Louis: Mosby, 1980.

Standards for Blood Banks and Transfusion Services (12th ed.). Arlington, Va.: American Association of Blood Banks, 1987.

Stites, D.P., Stobo, J.D., and Wells, J.V. (Eds.). *Basic and Clinical Immunology* (6th ed.). Norwalk, Conn.: Appleton & Lange, 1987.

Technical Manual of the American Association of Blood Banks (9th ed.). Philadelphia: Lippincott, 1985.

Tietz, N.W. (Ed.). *Fundamentals of Clinical Chemistry* (3rd ed.). Philadelphia: Saunders, 1987.

Washington, J.A. *Laboratory Procedures in Clinical Microbiology*. New York: Springer, 1981.

Weisbrot, I.M. *Statistics for the Clinical Laboratory*. Philadelphia: Lippincott, 1985.

Williams, W.J., et al. *Hematology* (3rd ed.). New York: McGraw-Hill, 1983.

Wintrobe, M.M. *Clinical Hematology* (8th ed.). Philadelphia: Lea & Febiger, 1981.